THE I
CAESAREAN
AND
VBAC GUIDE

by

TRACY DONEGAN

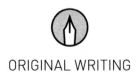

ORIGINAL WRITING

All rights reserved. No part of this publication may be reproduced
in any form or by any means—graphic, electronic or mechanical,
including photocopying, recording, taping or information storage and
retrieval systems—without the prior written permission of the author.

ISBN: 978-1-907179-68-6

A CIP catalogue for this book is available from the National Library.

Published by Original Writing Ltd., Dublin, 2010.
Printed by Cahills Printers Limited.

To Philip, Jack and Cooper

CONTENTS

INTRODUCTION

Welcome to The Irish Caesarean Birth and VBAC Guide. If you're reading this book then you may have just received the news that you may need a caesarean or you may be recovering from one. You may be an expectant Mum wondering if there is anything you can do to reduce your chances of having a surgical birth or how you can have a positive VBAC. The subheading of my book 'Choices and Challenges' aptly describes the experience of many Irish Mums trying to figure out the best option for them when it comes to birth choices around caesarean and vaginal birth after a caesarean. There's no doubt that planned surgery is stressful. Now combine emergency surgery with having a baby/becoming a Mother at the same time. I think it's safe to assume that the experts who annually list the top 10 stressors in life are most likely men!

As there are no national guidelines for Irish maternity care, standard policy in one unit may not be routine in another so doing a little bit of homework can really pay off in you and your baby having the safest and most positive experience possible.

As the Irish leader of ICAN (International Caesarean Awareness Network) I've provided support for hundreds of women around Ireland about to experience a surgical birth, recovering from surgical birth or wondering about their options for future pregnancies. If you're recovering from an unplanned caesarean, like most Mums you probably skipped the section on caesarean birth in your stack of pregnancy books (don't we all!). Antenatal classes tend to gloss over it or allocate it the same amount of time as breathing exercises – about 10 minutes. If you've read my first book The Better Birth Book you'll have seen the section on caesarean birth was titled 'Please Don't Skip Me!" When you're blissed out on pregnancy hormones you're not really thinking about having surgery – caesareans happen to other women – don't they? You may be thinking that you won't be one of 'those' women who are too posh to push etc etc and besides your caregiver isn't one of those scalpel happy Doctors you hear about in the newspapers.

Over the past few years working within the Irish maternity system one thing has become very clear. There is very little information available for Irish women about the Irish experience of caesarean birth.... From preparing for a planned positive caesarean birth ...to avoiding a caesarean, or recovering both physically and emotionally after an unplanned surgical birth. I hope this book will help you to prepare for a positive caesarean birth and make it easier to adjust to life after a caesarean with your newborn baby.

Also in this book you'll get tips from Irish mothers who have had caesarean births and those who have had VBAC (vaginal birth after caesarean). You'll learn ahead of time what these Mums wished they'd known before hand to make their experience a more positive one.

The guide is divided into 5 sections (no pun intended).

Chapter I   – What to Expect When Having a Caesarean

Chapter II   – Irish Caesarean Birth Stories

Chapter II   – Caesarean Birth – Why All The Fuss?

Chapter IV   – The Journey to VBAC

Chapter V   – Irish VBAC Birth Stories

CHAPTER I

▌ Caesarean History—So what have the Romans Ever Done for Us?

Legend has it that the term 'caesarean' came from Julius Caesar's caesarean birth but historians now consider that this is just a coincidence. JC's Mum lived long after his birth so it's very unlikely she had a caesarean . . . . but it's makes for a good story! Some writers suggest that in Roman times if a mother was near death during childbirth a caesarean would be performed. Roman King Numa Pompilius decreed it unlawful to bury an undelivered woman (715 BC). Anyone doing this would be guilty of causing the death of the child. From the 3rd Century BC -3rd Century AD ancient Jewish writings also mention caesarean births.

These days a caesarean birth is defined as the birth of a baby through an incision made in the abdomen and in to the uterus. A caesarean section is considered to be a relatively safe operation these days with the refinement of surgical skills, the development of antibiotics and more anaesthesia options so Mums can be awake while their baby is being born.

▌ What Usually Happens During a Caesarean?

(Note there may be slight differences in how your maternity unit practices)
Once the decision has been made to have an 'in labour' caesarean your Midwife will usually give you medication to neutralise the acid in your stomach. Depending on how serious the problem is your caesarean may need to happen immediately (also known as a crash caesarean) often this is the most frightening for Mums and their partners. Your baby needs to be born im-

mediately. An emergency caesarean is often not quite an emergency and the staff will have more time to prep you. At this point you may have a Midwife removing any nail polish you have on your fingers and toes (so the staff can keep an eye on your oxygen levels by checking how pink your nail beds are). You'll be put on a drip for surgery and your baby's heart rate will be monitored. If this is a crash caesarean you may suddenly have a team of staff around you immediately—try not to panic. You may have blood taken at this point also and a pair of TEDs stockings will be put on you (more on these later).

Staff will go through a check list with you about any allergies and have you remove any contact lenses, false teeth, hearing aids—any prosthesis. Have your partner bring your glasses so you can put them on immediately and see your newborn! (The teeth check is just in case you have to be intubated for a general anesthetic). Gummy smiles are adorable in newborns but you don't want to appear in all those lovely photos toothless!

You'll be asked to remove all of your jewellery—not because the Midwives want to have a gander at your solitaire engagement ring but because during surgery the surgeon may use an instrument (Diathermy) that uses an electrical current to cut tissue and reduce bleeding. If you are wearing metal jewellery which is in contact with your skin, you could end up with an electrical burn in the area of contact....so if you've any piercings in 'interesting' places....I'd suggest taking them out in the third trimester.

Shaving

In many cases your pubic hair will have a bit of a 'trim' as it *was* thought that it reduced infection and made access to the incision area easier but in more recent research it seems that shaving can cause tiny cuts in the skin and make infection more likely......if the choice is the momentary pain of a 'Hollywood' or an infected wound I know which one I'd prefer...

One concern that comes up again and again from Mums who had emergency caesareans was that nobody told them what was going on. Hopefully you'll have time for your Midwife to explain to you exactly what's going on and help calm your nerves.

Consent

You will sign a consent form for your surgery.

Fasting before a Planned Caesarean

It is recommended that you fast before a planned caesarean—during an emergency situation this is not possible (which is why you're given that medication to neutralise the acid in your stomach). If you're having a planned caesarean you may have been instructed to fast from midnight. If you're first on the theatre list then it's not such a problem but if you get bumped for an emergency you could be fasting for a long time and as you know a hungry Mum to be is not a happy Mum to be. New research from the UK suggests prolonged fasting causes problems in itself. The Royal College of Nursing (2005) UK national guideline recommends that patients can be given water and clear fluids 2 hrs before surgery and food can be given 6 hrs beforehand.

A Midwife or the emergency team will bring you to the theatre and your husband will wait outside and get gowned up and turned into your very own McDreamy (you always knew his talents were wasted in accounting). Once you've been given your spinal or epidural your partner will be brought in and he/she will sit up by your head. These days it's quite normal for partners to be present during a caesarean, provided you have an epidural and don't need a general anesthetic, which is rare. Check hospital policy on this.

▊ Anaesthesia

If you don't have an epidural already you'll be taken to theatre where an anaesthetist will inject the epidural into your back via a thin catheter if there is time. You'll feel a very cold liquid or spray on your on your back. You may have some stinging while the area of your back is numbed so the epidural or spinal injection can be inserted but this is usually momentary. You may have some shivering which can result both from the anaesthesia and the adrenaline. A catheter will be inserted into your bladder to drain your urine; this is generally done after the epidural has taken effect, so you won't feel anything. During this time focus on staying relaxed and slowing your breathing. In a non emergency caesarean there will be lots of staff casually walking around, setting everything up and possibly discussing last nights episode of Desperate Housewives. Although this is just an ordinary day for staff this is one of the biggest days of your life – you're about to meet your baby for the very first time. Don't let the staff's indifference dampen your enthusiasm and excitement on the biggest day of your life.

▊ Surgery

After your anaesthetic a curtain is hung between your neck and your lower body to create a sterile field. Sometimes it is possible to see the surgery in the mirrored overhead lights or an overhead TV screen. If you can see anything, try to focus on something else. Birth partners: help keep Mum positive and focus on the fact that you'll be meeting your new baby soon—remind her to slow her breathing down—you can help her by having her pace her breathing to yours. The anaesthetist will check to make sure you are numb before proceeding (in rare occasions the spinal doesn't work and Mum must be given a GA if your baby needs to be born immediately).

A horizontal incision is made with a scalpel, just above the pubic bone where the pubic hair begins; the Doctor cuts through the layers of skin, tissue, and muscle. You'll probably hear lots of odd noises like the suction machine. Birth partners: stay as calm as you can and focus on your partner's face, especially if blood makes you queasy.

You may feel a lot of pulling and tugging to dislodge the baby's head from the pelvis if your baby is well engaged. Most Mums report this as feeling very strange (but not painful). If your baby is in the head-down position, your baby is pulled backwards out of the pelvis (sometimes with forceps) and then by the head through the incision in the uterus (it's quite small). The baby's nose and mouth is sometimes suctioned to remove any amniotic fluid, mucous and/or meconium from the airway. The remainder of the baby's body is pulled from your uterus through the incision, taking care not to tear the uterine or abdominal incision wider.

Your baby is handed to a Midwife immediately who wraps your baby in a sterile sheet. She takes your baby to the warmer to check her over and dry and wrap her. There may be a paediatrician present. The theatres tend to be quite cold and babies can't regulate their own temperature so it's important to dry and warm your baby immediately. Dads can go to the warmer and see baby's first check. Assuming all is well, within minutes (but it feels like a lifetime for Mum) the Midwife or Dad will bring your new baby back to you for a kiss. In some circumstances your arms may have been strapped down so you can ask for your arms to be released so you can touch your baby. If there are any problems with your baby he/she may be taken to the intensive care unit for special care.

In many Irish maternity units Dad and baby go outside and then go up to the post natal ward to await Mum assuming baby is well. Sometimes Mums and babies are separated during this time much to the distress of the new mother. Check your hospital policy about keeping your baby with you in recovery. A great idea is for Dad to take a photo on his mobile and leave the phone with the nurse in the post op recovery area so Mum can see her new arrival. Dads you can give your baby skin to skin contact while you're waiting for Mum to come up from the recovery room. Pull the curtains around so you can have some privacy.

If You're Planning to Nurse Your Baby

While we're on the subject of skin to skin contact. Some Dads may be worried that your baby might be hungry in the time he's waiting for you to come to the post natal ward. If you're planning on breastfeeding there is no need to give your baby artificial milk in the meantime. Initiating breastfeeding with your baby within the first hour of birth is important—but there's no need to panic. Babies are born with enough fat reserves to get by quite well with tiny drops of colostrum which is the best food for your baby. You may have read stories about the tragedy in Haiti and the amazing stories of newborn babies being buried for up to a week and surviving with no food. Your baby may be a little unsettled—after all it's a big day for her too but your reassuring voice and some time to cuddle her will go along way. If you have concerns talk to your Midwife. If you are attending a hospital that has been awarded Baby Friendly status find out if you can have your baby with you in recovery. One of the criteria of your hospital being awarded Baby Friendly status is that Mums and babies are not separated.

Nearly There

A synthetic hormone is immediately injected to begin contractions of the uterus to help remove the placenta and reduce bleeding. Your Doctor will remove and examine it to ensure all pieces are intact and none of it is left behind in the uterus. Your uterus is then removed from your body (yes your uterus is now outside of your body) and placed on your stomach for the incision repair. One set of stitches is made in the wall of the uterus, then a second layer of stitches in the outer lining. The uterus is then pushed back through the abdominal incision and into your body. The staff will count the sponges, gauze and instruments to ensure none are left inside you (stranger things have happened...). The abdominal cavity is washed out with water to flush out any bacteria (to prevent infection) and check for bleeding. Your abdomen is then stitched and you are then moved to the recovery area. From the time of the epidural, you should see your baby in about 10 minutes, but the stitching up takes an additional 30–40 minutes and you may spend an hour or so in the recovery area with or without your baby. However if you've had a crash caesarean you may be in recovery for longer and are likely to feel quite woozy when you come around.

▌ The Importance of Skin to Skin Contact

Who's Your Daddy!

It's not always possible for you to have skin to skin contact with your newborn immediately after your caesarean but skin to skin with Dad has been shown to be very effective in soothing your newborn while you are in recovery. When Dad gets to the post natal ward pull the curtains and take off your shirt (what better reason to start using that gym membership you bought in January). Undress your baby to his nappy (your Midwife can help you with this if you're nervous) and hold your baby against your chest and cover both of you with a warm blanket. Or you can just have the Midwife place your baby up under your shirt. In a 2007 study the crying of infants in the skin-to-skin group decreased within 15 minutes of being placed skin-to-skin with Dad. These babies also became drowsy within 60 minutes after birth whereas babies left in the cots took nearly twice as long to nod off. Remember he just went from a calm, warm, quiet environment to bright lights, loud noises and strange people in a few minutes (and that's just Dad!). Having a cuddle together with Dad is a great way to start off.

Back on the post natal ward you'll have very sexy (not) TED stockings on to prevent blood clots forming—you may hear them referred to as 'clot socks'. When you don't move your legs for a long time the blood begins to pool in the veins and can cause clots to form. TEDs are usually a very flattering shade of white and have holes in the toes. You probably won't have seen this lovely lingerie at any Ann Summers parties.

Your Midwife will be by frequently to check your blood pressure, temperature, etc to make sure you are stable and recovering well. In some units you'll be given a PCA—(patient operated analgesia) so you can control your own pain medication dosage. Don't worry you can't overdose using it as it has a lockout system in place if you press the button too much.

Most Mums find this works very well. If you feel unwell—press the call button or ask for help from your neighbour. When the post natal ward is busy the squeaky wheel definitely gets the oil.

Within 24 hours, the urine catheter is removed and you are encouraged to stand and perhaps walk to the bathroom or shower, but you probably won't want to. But the sooner you're up and mobile the better. With a normal recovery you should be home in 5 days or less. If you think the scar may be infected you'll need antibiotics. Some Mums experience pain at the incision site intermittently for up to a year. Go easy on yourself and you're more likely to have a quick recovery.

▌ Nursing Your Baby after a Caesarean

Breastfeeding is not impossible after a caesarean but it can be more difficult. Don't force your baby to latch on as soon as you get to the ward—offer her skin to skin contact on your chest, talk to her and let your baby lead the way—your baby knows what to do! Many Mums report feeling very distant and drugged from the effects of the morphine pain relief so it's worth discussing alternative pain relief options with staff. Breastfeeding support is unpredictable in Irish hospitals and as I've already said it's definitely a case of the squeaky wheel gets the oil. Ask to see a Lactation Consultant especially if your baby has gone to special care so you can start using an electric pump to help bring your mature milk in while your baby is away from you.

Side-lying with your baby in bed with you to breastfeed will make breastfeeding much easier. Probably the hardest part of breastfeeding after a caesarean is just getting out of bed to get your baby. Ask the Midwife to bring your baby to you as often as you need to nurse him or have someone stay with you as much as possible during the first few days at the hospital to help pass the baby to you. Surgery can affect how quickly your mature milk comes in too, so don't be surprised if your milk takes a little longer to come in after a caesarean. (It's usually two or three days for a normal vaginal birth.) Even if you feel you don't have any milk your baby is getting all he needs from the tiny drops of liquid gold (colostrum). Your newborns stomach is about the size of a Milky Moo mint so they need very little in those first few days.

Adapted with permission from KellyMom.com

First Nursing After a Caesarean Birth

If possible, the time immediately after your baby is born is a great time to start breastfeeding. You will still be under the effects of the spinal/epidural and probably not yet feeling any discomfort. You will likely have to nurse lying on your back, because of the epidural or ask your Midwife to help you sit up a little bit. Since one arm will probably have a drip in it, it may get a little tricky. Try positioning baby lying face down across your breasts (similar to cradle hold, but baby is higher up and away from your incision, and Mum is lying flat). When nursing in this position with a newborn, have someone nearby to make sure baby's nose doesn't get blocked, since you both may be groggy from the meds. Have your partner or a Midwife help position the baby, and use lots of pillows around you to help with support.

Nurse early and often. Ideally, you'll want to put your baby to breast within the first hour, but definitely no later than the first 4-6 hours. Studies show that when time to breast is longer than this, babies have more difficulty breastfeeding and engorgement is more severe. If something prevents the baby from being put to breast within the 4-6 hours, you should begin pumping with a hospital-grade breast pump.

Ask to see the Lactation Consultant. Breastfeeding at least every 2 hours during the day with a night time span no longer than 4 hours is highly recommended--you're aiming for 8—10 feedings per 24 hours during the early weeks. As long as baby is nursing well, there should be no need for any supplements of any kind (i.e. artificial milk or sugar water).

Nursing positions

Once you can turn over, try turning to one side and nursing in a side-lying position. Have your partner or a nurse help you with positioning pillows.

Another position that may be more comfortable is the football hold. Sit somewhat upright in the bed and place the baby on a pillow, between your arm and your side, with your hand cupping the underside of his head.

You may find at first that it's difficult to find a "comfortable" nursing position. Try experimenting as much as possible to get the most comfortable position, and don't hesitate to ask for help getting positioned from your partner, Midwives, or the hospital Lactation Consultant. Whichever position works best, make sure the baby's tummy is towards you. You might want to bring a few extra pillows from home (or a nursing pillow) as hospital pillows are pretty small and flat.

Many Mums find the side-lying position the most comfortable during the first day or so. It's an easy way to nurse and rest at the same time. Using a small blanket, or pillow—even a rolled up towel—can help protect your incision while you nurse lying down.

Below are step-by-step instructions on getting into the side-lying position (in a hospital bed) after a caesarean section:

• Begin with the bed in a flat position and side rails up.

• Use extra pillows behind the mother's back for extra support.

• Carefully roll to one side while grasping the side rail and relaxing the abdominal muscles. Move slowly to avoid strain.

• To protect the incision from the baby's kicking, cover the abdomen with a small pillow or towel.

• Place a pillow between the legs to minimize the strain on the stomach muscles.

• Lean back into the pillows behind the back.

• When using side-lying position, baby should be placed on his side, facing your body, chest to chest, so he doesn't have to turn his head to nurse. Baby's feet should be drawn in close to your body with his head either lying on the bed, or on your arm, whichever feels most comfortable to you. You can either roll your body forward to latch, or pull the baby toward you.

Avoid Supplements

Be sure to let the hospital staff know they shouldn't give any supplemental bottles or pacifiers/soothers, as these artificial nipples can cause problems with breastfeeding. If you are told that supplements are medically necessary, request that they be given via cup or feeding syringe rather than a bottle to avoid the risk of nipple preference. A baby has to work harder on the breast and like most of us we'll go with the easier option.

▊ When Will My Mature Milk Come In?

Colostrum is your early milk and is soon followed by your mature milk. Your breasts can produce milk from as early as the 2nd trimester. The abrupt hormonal shift that occurs at the separation of the placenta from the uterus is what signals your milk to come in. Your body will get the same signal whether you have a caesarean or vaginal birth. Mums who have stressful births (caesarean or vaginal) tend to have their milk come in a little bit later.

Your milk may come in anywhere from day 2 to day 6 (usually around days 2-3). If your milk is slow coming in, try not to worry, but put baby to breast as often as possible and stay in contact with your Lactation Consultant so she can monitor how baby is doing. Your baby does very well on colostrum alone in the early days, as nature intended.

▊ To Encourage an Abundant Milk Supply:

Nurse as soon after birth as possible. If something prevents the baby from being put to breast within the 4-6 hours, you should begin pumping with a hospital-grade breast pump. Get the okay from your Doctor/Midwife ahead of time to nurse your baby in the recovery room—this shouldn't be a problem unless you or baby are having medical problems.

Nurse frequently. Breastfeed your baby at least every 2 hours (from beginning of nursing to beginning of the next nursing) during the day, with no more than 4 hours between nursings at night. Let your baby tell you when he's interested. You're aiming for at least 10-12 nursings within 24 hours. More frequent nursing results in greater milk production at one week and thereafter. Although this might seem like a lot consider how many times a day you eat or drink anything—even a cup of tea or a few sips from your water bottle. If we're being honest with ourselves you'll see that normal healthy adults who aren't actively trying to lose weight or put it on will eat/drink something around 10—12 times a day. Make a list of every single thing you ate yesterday and you'll see what I mean—keep in mind that your baby is trying to double his weight in 6 months.

Avoid unnecessary supplements. Avoid supplementing your baby with anything (formula, water, etc) unless it is medically indicated. Supplementing will do two things—missing feedings will reduce breast stimulation and milk removal (both needed to increase milk supply), and babies who are supplemented tend to need to eat again later than if they had nursed—so again you're losing much-needed nursing time.

Ensure that baby is nursing well. If baby is not latching well and transferring milk well, then it can affect milk supply and the speed that your milk comes in.

Going Home

If all is going well, some Mums prefer to ask for an earlier discharge so they are not at the hospital for an extended length of time. If you do this, be sure that you have some help at home, and try to get as much rest and nourishment as possible—especially fluids. Do see if there is a Lactation Consultant at the hospital (or another local Lactation Consultant with a private practice) who will make at least a couple of home visits to be sure all is going well with breastfeeding, and help you (if necessary)to fine-tune positioning and latching.

Get help around the house postpartum. If possible, have your partner take a few days to several weeks off work (as much as you can afford!) to help out. You won't be up to housework at ALL at first. Even accomplishing basic tasks for your own and your baby's needs will be tough. This is major surgery. Your body will need time to recover. If taking time off is not an option for your partner, look into getting others to help. Do you have friends or family who can check in on you? Someone to help with the washing, dishes and cooking? Can you pay a professional to clean up once a week (this will make you feel better). Consider hiring a post natal doula to come and help you in these first few challenging but exciting weeks.

▓ Staying Comfortable After a Caesarean

You will need some help in the first few days; staff are often busy, but do not be afraid to ask.

- Take it slowly. You'll probably feel like you've been hit by a bus the next day especially if you've laboured and then had an emergency caesarean. Be kind to yourself. Just getting out of bed is going to be very painful in the beginning. The Midwives will want you up and about quickly; they're not doing it to torture you— it's important for you to be up and mobile to prevent blood clots. Those first few steps are going to be hard and you will need help. If you've never had surgery before, it can be a shock how your body reacts and how much it takes out of you. Take baby steps and don't rush yourself. Mums are often surprised to learn that they have to take care of their newborn immediately following a caesarean due to the policy of rooming in. Although the policy in itself promotes bonding and breastfeeding with understaffing at night and at the weekends it can be the cause of incredible trauma for post caesarean mothers when they can't physically get out of bed to pick up their screaming newborn. If you'd just had your appendix out you wouldn't be expected to take care of a newborn infant while you recover but after a caesarean it's a very different ball game.

- Take the drugs. Even if you are breastfeeding, your Doctors and Midwives will still urge you to take pain relief. You'll feel better and you'll be more motivated to stick with the breastfeeding (avoid Morphine if breastfeeding). The actual amount of medications that will reach your breastmilk and your baby are minimal and quite safe but be sure that your caregiver knows that you are breastfeeding. You will need those medications to help you during those first few weeks in order to walk, sleep, etc.

- Let others help you. Swallow your pride and let your partner, family or friends help you with the house and caring for the baby. Even a simple task like climbing into bed can make you feel like a 90-year-old.

- Keep your necessities close. Having necessary items such as nappies, wipes, tissues, mobile phone, paper towels, remote control, pain medications, bottles, nipple cream, etc. close at hand will help tremendously. Having them next to you will help keep you from having to continuously get up and down or move from room to room.

- Pulling to a sitting position. Those tummy muscles that you once took for granted will be of no use to you for the first few weeks following your operation. To pull yourself from a lying position to a sitting one, be sure to either have someone help you or use something like the back of the couch to pull yourself up gently. Another good trick if you are lying on a couch or bed is to try gently rolling off it (assuming it is not too high off the ground) to the floor and then pull yourself up using a sturdy object such as a table or a nightstand.

- Avoid stairs. If at all possible; avoid climbing stairs for at least the first week. If your room is upstairs, set up camp downstairs on the couch.

- Create a pillow splint. Laughing, sneezing, coughing or taking deep breaths those first few days will be extremely painful. If you need to do any of those things, take a soft pillow and press it gently to your abdomen.

- Avoid greasy foods and carbonated drinks: Once your bowels begin working properly after surgery, you will be extremely gassy. Gas bubbles will wreak havoc on your sensitive insides. Be sure to avoid anything that will only irritate your bowels further. Ask your Midwife about warm Peppermint water to sip on—you'll probably let rip for Ireland after it but it can really help with those colicky sensations.

- Keep checking your incision: You might not want to look at it, but keep an eye on it. Your Doctor will advise you on what he/she would like you to do to keep the area clean. Report any inflammation, redness or discharge. Some New Zealand Midwives use Manuka honey on caesarean section wounds because of it's high antibacterial qualities. You can also wash the area with a blend of warm water, Tea Tree oil and Lavender oil to prevent infection. (Tea Tree oil has been shown to be effective against MRSA)

- Invest in a caesarean belt to give your abdomen extra support while you heal.

Emotional Care after a Caesarean

Depending on the circumstances of your caesarean section, you will most likely have conflicting emotions surrounding the event. Top it off with the normal post-partum hormonal freefall and you may feel like an emotional wreck. Talk to someone you trust about how you feel, or talk with other mothers who have experienced the same things. Get in touch with your local ICAN group. Don't be afraid to cry and don't feel ashamed of your feelings and don't let any one tell you how you 'should' be feeling. Often well meaning friends will tell you to focus on the fact that you have a healthy baby but that doesn't take away from the feelings of grief that many women experience after an unplanned caesarean birth.

You may feel shocked, robbed, angry, disappointed, or maybe relieved after your caesarean. For some women a caesarean birth is physically a huge handicap for a few weeks but emotionally they are fine. For other women an unplanned caesarean birth can be not just physically but emotionally debilitating too. We all interpret events differently and each woman's reaction is a personal experience. Many women who have caesareans suffer in silence because society expects them to "just be happy you have a healthy baby." Friends and family say, "Be grateful; a hundred years ago you both would have died." Caesarean scars are seen as well as unseen. The unseen scars can take longer to heal.

We know from research that a mother never forgets the day she gave birth. A Mum's satisfaction of her baby's birth isn't usually about pain, or interventions but how she was treated by the staff. Were you treated like a Queen or an inconvenience? Were you treated with dignity or as an interruption? With the growing number of caesareans is it possible that staff becoming desensitized to the enormity of this event on the mother?

▌ Coping with the Emotional Aftermath of a Caesarean—*Adapted from Plus Sized Pregnancy with Permission.*

Women have a wide range of emotional responses after a caesarean. Some are devastated by it, some love it, some are disappointed but okay with it, some feel 'rescued' by it, and some seem fine at first only to experience delayed grieving later. There are many factors that can influence how a woman experiences and interprets a caesarean emotionally.

▌ Planned Caesarean vs. Unplanned Caesarean

Whether or not the caesarean was planned is often (but not always) a factor in how you experience your caesarean and the aftermath.

If your caesarean was planned a head of time generally your physical and emotional recovery is faster than a Mum who is rushed to theatre with panicked staff ignoring her pleas to know what's going on. You've had time to adjust....to plan...to be in a positive mind frame for what's ahead. You will generally be in good shape and not exhausted after a difficult labour.

▌ Experience of Labour

Another factor that strongly influences a woman's experience of caesarean birth is how her labour went—especially how she was treated.

If a woman experienced a relatively easy labour but a situation suddenly occurred where a caesarean became necessary, some women feel robbed of the culmination of what they had been working towards. These women tend to adjust fairly quickly and are often able to navigate recovery easily enough. They usually do not face future pregnancies or births with much fear of labour, just the fear of the recurrence of the specific complication recurring. Once they get past the stage where the complication occurred, they generally do very well. Sometimes they do experience the complication recurring, but with a more favourable resolution, and then they are fine.

On the other hand, sometimes women who have had a sudden caesarean due to an emergency during labour are traumatized by the suddenness of how things changed, the unpredictable nature of labour, and a sense of fear over this volatility. The quick action that sometimes must be taken because of complications often does not leave time for women to adjust emotionally; they may feel like their bodies and emotions have been hijacked. Sometimes staff just don't have time to talk to you in an emergency to explain what's going on. In subsequent labours, even if everything is going well, they may fear another sudden 'hijacking' by a complication, and often need a lot of reassurance that all is going well. Again, once they are past the point where the previous complication occurred, they can often relax a bit more.

Women who experienced a very difficult and painful labour before their caesarean occurred often see the caesarean as a welcome release from the pain they experienced. These are often the women who 'loved' their caesareans, as to them it was a

release or a rescue from a difficult situation. To go from an im-
mense amount of pain with little or no progress to the numbness of caesarean anaesthesia may feel like a real blessing, and
to have the immediate gratification of having it all over and
holding that precious little one in their arms sooner rather than
later is an understandable joy.

Many women in this position logically therefore see their anaesthetist or consultant as rescuer and hero. Ironically, many of
these difficult labours were actually caused by the labour management policies of the Doctors, who were then able to ride in
on their white horse to 'rescue' the woman from the problem
the Doctors had created in the first place. Women in this situation usually divide into two camps---those who staunchly keep
seeing their Doctors as white knight rescuers, and those whose
heroes get knocked from the pedestals when they find out that
the actions of their Doctors may have caused their caesareans
in the first place.

This is a particularly difficult emotional transition. A woman
may be 'fine' with her caesarean at first because she saw it as
a rescue from a difficult situation or a lifesaving measure for
herself or her baby. If she finds out later that the Doctor actually caused or greatly added to the problem that she had to
be rescued from (or even worse, put her baby's life in danger
through his actions), that transition from loving the caesarean
to feeling betrayed by it can be particularly harrowing. This is
often seen when Mums request copies of their birth notes and
have a chance to sit down and understand why things happened
and if their caesarean was really necessary. If she idolized her
Doctor/hero only to have him fall from the pedestal in a big way
later on, then all of her beliefs about medicine and childbirth
are shaken to their core. These women often start out 'fine' with
their caesarean but have a very difficult time healing emotionally once they truly understand their prior labour and birth.

Women who are induced, have a long and painful labour, and
end in an unanticipated caesarean can also have a particularly

hard emotional recovery. A caesarean after a long difficult induction can be particularly challenging physically, and induction drugs often have long-term physical effects too. We know that inductions for non medical reasons bump up your chances of a caesarean by nearly 40%.

A typical scenario is a Mum is told that her baby is big so an induction is planned the induction fails and the woman is now convinced that her baby was in fact too big but it was the induction that failed—not the mother's body.... in many cases there would have been a different outcome had the Mum gone into labour spontaneously.

Pitocin, for example, can cause significant swelling and oedema in the mother, which may impact breastfeeding supply, make it difficult and painful to walk, and be very uncomfortable to deal with. Babies who have experienced labours with lots of drugs and pain medications can be jaundiced, drowsy, and 'out of it' at first, then fussy later on. All of these physical factors tend to make emotional recovery much more difficult as well.

Adding to the difficulty of physical and emotional recovery after a difficult induction is the fear factor. Some inductions are so difficult that women develop a tremendous fear about labour. They can feel traumatized by how hard it was and how much pain they went through. Many have great anxiety about going through labour again because their only experience of labour was such an unnaturally strong and painful one. As a result, many choose an elective caesarean for their next birth in order to avoid a recurrence of such a difficult labour, not knowing (or not being able to trust) that labour doesn't have to be that painful and hard. In Scandinavian studies over half of women who have post birth counselling after a difficult birth ending in caesarean often change their minds and decide to go for VBAC. This kind of psychological counselling is not freely available in Ireland.

▌ Experience of Surgery and Recovery

What happens during surgery and recovery also influences a woman's perception about her caesarean.

If the surgery was experienced as a relief after a long and very difficult labour, many women feel 'rescued' by it, and may always want to have a caesarean in the future. If they have never experienced an uncomplicated vaginal birth and have no comparison of how much easier a vaginal birth is to recover from, then they have no standard by which to measure a surgical recovery. Therefore, if their surgical recovery was unremarkable, these women are inclined to think of a caesarean as 'no big deal'.

On the other hand, if surgery was difficult or traumatic in any way, a woman's perception of her caesarean is understandably going to be more negative, and her emotional recovery afterwards more difficult. For example, some women have experienced a lack of complete anaesthesia coverage during their caesareans, which can be absolutely devastating emotionally and physically. This type of experience has long-term effects on feelings and fears about birth and surgery, and is a very difficult issue to heal from. It also can involve Post-Traumatic Stress Disorder. True recovery often involves going back and revisiting and reprocessing the experience and the difficulty of doing that can keep women from healing for a long time. However, emotional recovery is possible, and the experience can often be a potent healing influence.

If a woman's physical recovery is difficult or involved after a caesarean, then her emotional recovery will also likely be affected. Since larger women are more at risk for infections and wound separations after a caesarean, this can be an issue for them (although it should be noted that average-sized women can encounter problems too!). If a woman's incision site will not close, develops an infection or pockets of fluid, then she may need long-term nursing care. Sometimes women even need to be re-admitted to the hospital for additional surgery on the site. Caesareans also increase the risk for postpartum health problems like gallstones, appendicitis, ectopic pregnancy, painful scar adhesions, and possibly infertility. If you experienced problems like this, it's understandable not appreciating the caesarean, or having difficulty recovering emotionally afterwards!

▌ Treatment by Staff

As mentioned earlier—how you were treated by the medical staff during your labour, during your caesarean, and during your recovery also influences your opinions about caesareans and your emotional recovery from them. When you entered the hospital did you feel like you were in a supportive environment surrounded by encouraging friends? Or did you feel like an inconvenience?

If the staff were consistently helpful, nurturing, empathetic and considerate towards your feelings, this goes a long way towards helping you towards physical and emotional healing. You may still experience disappointment over your caesarean but probably won't be as deeply traumatized by it.

On the other hand, if staff were uncaring, cold, distant, judgmental, or abusive during labour, the caesarean, or recovery, you're highly likely to find your caesarean traumatic and have some difficulties recovering emotionally. Although we would like to think that all hospital staff are caring and considerate, some staff can be very insensitive. It's nothing personal—but someone can just be having a bad day and you get the brunt of it.

As you read some of the less positive caesarean birth stories later you might understand better how some women can find their caesareans deeply traumatic, and carry long-term emotional wounds from them.

▌ Necessity of Surgery

How necessary the surgery was is also a very important factor in how you'll perceive your caesarean.

If the surgery truly saved your life or the life of your baby, your feelings about it will be different from a woman who was felt she was bullied into surgery unnecessarily or not given any options. For some women, knowing their surgery was necessary helps them recover emotionally without a great deal of regret. Their disappointment about the caesarean may be overshadowed by gratitude that surgery was possible and available, and that they and their child are alive to tell about the experience.

However, even when surgery is truly necessary or life-saving, some Mums still mourn the loss of their ideal birth and the changes that had to occur due to circumstances. These women are often told "at least you have a healthy baby" and that they should be thankful for the life-saving surgery, but often find this an extremely frustrating and disempowering statement.

Of course it is true that a healthy baby is the top priority, and if the caesarean was truly necessary, then we can be grateful intellectually for the procedure. It is insulting to suggest otherwise. However, even when the surgery was necessary, a woman often needs to mourn the birth she wished she could have or was not allowed to have, and to acknowledge the difficulty of having major surgery. Having major abdominal surgery right before taking care of a needy and high-maintenance newborn is not easy! Most women would not choose to adopt a baby and bring it home on the day they had their gallbladders out, yet people routinely dismiss the physical impact of caesarean surgery on the mother. And for some women, to be told that they have no right to mourn the loss of their ideal birth in addition to the physical invasiveness and burden of surgery is insult added to injury.

If women who truly needed a caesarean can still find it distressing, imagine the bitterness and intensity of mourning in women who find out that their caesarean was unnecessary or could have been prevented! Depending on which hospital you are attending about half of all caesareans in Ireland are estimated to be 'unnecessary', and as we'll discuss later, are often caused by the management policies of the hospitals themselves. When a woman realizes this difficult and invasive experience could have been avoided, the anger and bitterness she experiences often makes emotional healing difficult. On the other hand, if she is able to channel this anger into empowerment, this may also propel her into great action and healing in birth issues and in life.

There are also women who really don't care how their babies arrive in the world, who see caesarean birth and vaginal birth as truly interchangeable, and simply do not see a caesarean as any big deal. They are often able to adapt and 'go with the flow' easily and don't care how they give birth, or just don't see a birth experience as important and would just as soon get it over with. Some of these women have had a difficult time imagining themselves actually giving birth vaginally, and so are not disappointed if it does not happen. To them, it doesn't really make much difference either way.

On the other hand, if a woman strongly believes that birth is a natural occurrence and dreams of a birth that is totally natural and medication-free, a caesarean often shakes her belief in the safety and naturalness of birth, and shakes her trust in her body. Women who strongly desire a totally natural birth yet experience a caesarean often have a difficult time integrating that experience.

Women who had a strong ideal of birth beforehand that was not fulfilled in reality also often have a hard time mourning the birth that they wanted and didn't get. There is nothing wrong with a strong vision of birth, but it is important to be able to be flexible and adapt because birth is not always predictable. These women have to find a way to maintain their vision of birth but be able to 'go with the flow' if things happen differently, and to encompass into their vision a way to have a positive birth if a problem makes different choices necessary. Mourning their caesarean often helps these women find that compromise of vision with flexibility.

Some women see birth as a pass/fail test. They are often high achievers who place a high priority on 'doing things right' and doing a good job at all times. Being 'out of control' during the most intense part of labour may frighten them, and the thought of 'failing' at labour may have them petrified. Experiencing a caesarean is often devastating to these women, but if they let it, the experience can help them find the ability to release control and embrace the uncertainty of life.

Women experience their caesareans in vastly different ways, depending on the beliefs and fears they brought to the birth, how well they were treated during labour and birth, how the surgery and recovery went for them, and how necessary the surgery really was. Although these generalizations about women's experiences are obviously a bit over-simplified, they do contain many truths about how and why women respond so differently to what seems on the surface to be the same experience. Remember, no judgments are implied here; these are simply observations that may help explain why different people experience the same incident so differently.

Did you find yourself, your beliefs, or your situation described at all above? Many women who read these observations will see themselves, perhaps in multiple ways. Other women may not see themselves at all.

Take some time to consider to yourself how you have responded to your caesarean, and what factors might have influenced that response. Don't be judgmental; simply observe your influences and reflect on them. This may contain some of the keys to help you towards healing after your caesarean.

You are not wrong or crazy or neurotic or wimpy or selfish for feeling the way that you feel. Expert Lynn Madsen writes:

You cannot expect every person around you to understand your feelings completely, but you can ask them to acknowledge and respect the fact that you have these feelings. You can't expect everyone around you to be in constant mourning with you over your birth, but you should be able to expect them to acknowledge that you were hurt, that you have the right to your feelings, and to give you space for the mourning and healing that you need to do.

Sometimes, you simply have to tell friends that they may not fully understand why you are so upset over your birth experience, but they do need to understand that you ARE upset by it, and that they need to respect that. Sometimes, you have to instruct them on what you need----a listening but non-judgmental ear, someone to bounce ideas off of, a helper to take the baby for an hour or two so you can take time to really grieve, or whatever. Sometimes, strong or repeated conflict is an indication that you are having boundary issues with someone, and that you need to become more assertive and set more strict limits with that person. Occasionally, you simply have to declare the subject off-limits with certain people, and if necessary get up and leave.

On the other hand, it's important to understand and respect that other people have different views of birth. You don't need to convert everyone around you into your point of view about birth; if you want them to respect your point of view, you have to respect that they may completely disagree with you. As Madsen notes, "With the emotionally loaded subject of birth, differences in philosophy and practice make for volatile encounters. Without the agreement to disagree with respect, primary relationships such as marriage, parent-daughter, and friend-ships can be torn apart." Remember, their beliefs in different birth values than yours does NOT invalidate your beliefs. Don't be threatened by someone else's beliefs, just agree to disagree.

However, some people may never 'get it.' They may have too much of their own 'stuff' in the way, they may have their own agendas about birth, or they may not be willing or able to really acknowledge and deal with someone else's pain. Madsen urges women to seek support for their healing journey from sources where they will get it. Don't keep looking for understanding from people who are not capable of giving it; instead seek out sources where you are more likely to find understanding or a sympathetic ear. Seek out many different types of resources, as one may not be able to provide you with all the support you need. Combine resources as needed in order to meet all of your various requirements.

▌ Mental Preparation for your Caesarean Birth

It's well documented that the less anxious a patient is before surgery the more positive the experience and interestingly enough the quicker their recovery. (I use the term 'patient' within the medical context of having surgery—not within the realms of normal birth when a Mum is not sick). Most people going in to surgery are going to have something 'fixed' a Mum going in to caesarean surgery is also contending with the fact that she's about to become a mother in a matter of minutes. Double the stress! Going in to surgery it's so important to be as calm as possible. It's even more important to remain calm if your cae-sarean is unexpected. When you're in a state of high anxiety your blood pressure rises, your pulse rate increases and your immune system is suppressed. Your body redirects blood to the skeletal muscles (arms and legs) as part of the fight or flight re-sponse. It's simple biology—cell growth/healing is determined by the amount of blood the organ receives but when you are in a panic the blood is shunted from the uterus as it's not a defensive organ unlike your arms and legs. This reduces blood flow not just to the muscle of the uterus but also to your baby.

The more stress you are under the more chronically you suppress the growth/healing mechanism. The same hormones that are excreted during stress are the same hormones that are used by organ transplant teams to shut down the immune system so that the body won't reject the organ. Preparing for your positive caesarean needs to involve a shift from fear to calm so that you are stacking the odds in your favour of a quick recovery with the minimum of post surgery complications so you can have a more enjoyable start to parenthood with your new born baby.

One of the quickest ways to counter the fight/flight response is to slow down your breathing which is easier said then done when a dozen staff descends upon you, machines are beeping and alarms screaming. Discuss this with your birth partner ahead of time as part of your birth preparation. Their job is to keep you calm and focused. If you have a relaxation CD that you've been using during your pregnancy put it on. If not have your partner talk to you and encourage you to focus on your breathing—nothing else but your breathing and meeting your baby. Let the staff do their job while you do yours—staying calm.

Chapter II

▍ Caesarean Birth Stories in Ireland

- I had my section 8 months ago and I have to say I'm glad I had one. (I was not looking forward to all the labour pains!!) My baby was breech for the last 8 weeks and I'm also a type 1 diabetic so I was glad cause this was my first baby and I didn't know what to expect. Don't get me wrong it was scary, but I felt no pain during the section, and I couldn't have gotten better care, the nurses and Doctor were fabulous. I spent first night in public ward which was awful because I obviously couldn't move and the baby was awake all night cause of all the other babies crying, the nurses were run off their feet so I was left most of the night trying to rock my baby from bed. I got moved to a private room the second day and that was great. Pain was bad for first two days but I had plenty of pain killers. Once I had a shower on second day felt much better. Overall I have to say I felt I got great care and hope that if I have another baby I would try to have another section.

- I wish I knew about having a caesarean that the risk of nerve damage was high and I would not have feeling in my left leg again. I think most people know what goes on in theatre but not the physical and mental healing that goes on afterwards. Having to learn to get out of bed a certain way...cough in a certain way.....even trying to go to the toilet. The surgery pains. Mentally I found it more difficult. How was I going to cuddle my toddler? I was going to have to rely on others for the first time in my adult life. If I have another baby what about the scar? There's just so many questions.

- I had an emergency section last September. I was a week overdue and was in very early labour—had a show, couldn't feel as much movement as usual, put on a monitor—the Midwives and Doctor not happy with foetal heart rate, so off to theatre. I think people should be told that a c section is actually NOT THAT BAD! It's the aftermath that's the problem.

- I was so convinced I'd be having a natural birth, I was even going to go without an epidural, so a c section was a total shock—I hadn't even bothered to read about it in any of my many books! Instead both my baby and I ended up drugged up to the eyeballs... The recovery didn't take that long—although the day afterwards, I felt that I was going to split in half when I tried to get out of bed—a lot of it is psychological.

- I wish I'd know sooner that I would definitely end up having a section and therefore not spend 8 months planning a wonderful homebirth. Due to the lack of anomaly scanning equipment in all hospitals, I had a baby born with limb body wall complex. This can be detected as early as 14wks. I had a scan at 10wks and 19wks and was told all was fine. I went into labour at 36wks with a breech presentation, so a section was inevitable. Our girl was born with external organs, very under developed lungs, a missing foot and the cord was only 8" long in total. As a result she only lived for 2hrs. I just wished our hospital system utilized their equipment and procedures better. Yes, sections save lives, but are so many necessary? If the budget was spend on educating women on mind and body birth preparation, in more comfortable surroundings with genuine Midwives, maybe they could save 1000's from less caesarean sections. Therefore update their scanning equipment for the whole country. Not just city hospitals

Annette

- My birth experience was very traumatic and I'm still trying to come to terms with what happened. I didn't even go into half of what happened to me as it was a nightmare from start to finish.

  I had an emergency caesarean which resulted in a uterine rupture and led to post partum haemorrhage. I lost so much blood I had to have a blood transfusion as a result. I consider myself and my baby to be very blessed to have survived of course but the whole thing still stays with me.

  I guess there was no way I could have been prepared for this regardless of what I read beforehand. Though I do think they should forewarn you the awful effect the drugs can potentially have on you afterwards and make people aware of this. I feel that not everyone's system can take the sheer volume they pump into you. I had a very severe reaction to one particular drug. I didn't know what was wrong with me and really thought I was losing my mind it caused myself, my baby and my family unnecessary strain and huge stress seeing me in such a state. I also feel the care in the hospital is not adequate in that you are expected to take care of your baby the same as a lady who gave birth naturally which is next to impossible when you are in pain whatever way you turn, immobile and bed ridden with a catheter. The aftercare for c-sections is practically non existent and they send you off with your new baby having gone through major abdominal surgery and you just have to get on with it. It's very different to a natural birth with a tough recovery period and you are left with a huge scar that can potentially affect your body image. I found it extremely difficult being in so much pain trying to look after a baby and breastfeed at the same time in hospital but especially at home. I felt I couldn't cope initially and was inconsolable at times. My partner and family had to do a lot simply because I couldn't. I couldn't even lift my baby for weeks. On leaving the hospital I was handed a leaflet on how to get in and out of bed etc. but absolutely nothing prepared me for the pain, my wound opening up, two infections, persistent bleeding from the incision, haematomas which I had to get removed in my senses twice, and at times severe pain that I am still experiencing over three months on. I had absolutely no inkling that anything close to this could happen to me. I've since had 3 courses of antibiotics to treat infections, swabs, an ultrasound, an MRI scan, and I'm still in pain….and no one can tell me why.

Honestly, at times I wonder how I am expected to live with this degree of pain and when I can feel normal again. If it wasn't for my beautiful baby I don't know how I'd get through it. I feel it's a great idea to allow women to share their experience as no one really is ever prepared for what could happen. Also to let others know that they are not on their own with how they are feeling.

- My problem is that my daughter was covered in meconium and had a collapsed lung so ended up in special care having a chest drain. That traumatised me a lot. She was there for a week. Things I wish I'd known are that it takes longer for your milk to come in. I was desperate to breastfeed and although I combined fed for 6 weeks, it didn't really work for me—probably I now think due to stress and also anxiety about how much she was getting, blood sugar etc—from special care. I don't think my milk ever really came in enough. Also I also probably overdid it on the morphine at the beginning which probably had an impact on the breast feeding. I wish someone could have given me some definitive advice on this. Also I have a 'special' place in my heart for the Midwife who handed me a replacement pair of those blood clot socks after my first shower and said if I needed a hand putting them on to let her know…. Another Midwife couldn't believe she had left a woman with a c section wound to try to put on the socks on her own! Anyway, there was a time I could have gone on about this forever but I think women should be told that a c section doesn't have to be that bad. My recovery was absolutely fine, and very very quick. The scar is unremarkable. Also, although Doctors are often criticised for being too quick to section, in cases such as mine they don't have a choice in my opinion. Baby too high up to take blood sample, I could see and hear her heart rate dipping alarmingly every time I had a very mild contraction—I wouldn't have wanted them to do anything else. But it can be very very stressful afterwards, particularly if there are implications for the baby. It's only now, that a friend has had a very smooth natural delivery that I'm even feeling aggrieved that I didn't have a chance to do that...

That being said, even though I had wanted as natural a birth as possible, when I was going up and down to feed my baby in special care, I'd see women walking the corridors in labour, and a teeny tiny very guilty little part of me thought "phew, thank god I didn't have to go through that!"

- Thanks for including caesarean section birth stories I often feel that this is completely ignored.

  I was to have a section as my baby was breech. My consultant said as he would let me try for a vaginal birth if I wanted however as it was my first we decided that section was better option. He then said that he would not section me until due date to give my baby all the time to turn. I had to go into CUMH night before the scheduled date as I was having pains was sent home told it was Braxton hicks. I went in again next morning early pains getting worse never examined waited all day for bed was given premed by a student who couldn't tell me what it was so I stupidly took it. I went to surgery at 7 pm. The anaesthetist was horrible to me and even my consultant reprimanded him. No Midwife spoke to me in theatre.Two Filipino nurses spoke Filipino over me in recovery. The good side was I got to see Roisin being born on camera and was shown her straight away. I had to remind them to bring in my husband.

  I felt it was all a big rush and very impersonal. Post op I asked to breastfeed in recovery and was tutted—they gave out that they would have to turn me over. I am so glad I insisted though. Back on ward my baby was taken for the night and I had to ring to bring her back to me. There was a mix up over my analgesia so ended up with paracetamol only for 48 hrs. I got no Difene, PCA pump, Tramadol or even Solpadol until a fab student Midwife sorted it out she was also great with breastfeeding when my baby got jaundice. I had my baby on Thursday night was home Monday and got the winter vomiting bug on Tuesday evening (turns out there was an outbreak in hospital)

To top it all off my baby got MRSA. I hate to say it but it was a bad experience I can't say terrible as I have my healthy happy baby.

- I was induced on the Thurs morn and had emergency section on the Sat morning about 10am! I was really quite fortunate because although I lost a lot of blood during the operation I was only borderline blood transfusion candidate so I had to take iron tablets for months! One thing I do wish I had known was though that I took the morphine for two days but wasn't given the baby at night time! That was grand the first night but the second I got very upset because I wasn't told that was what would happen if I had the morphine.... yet I had full care of the baby during the day while also on morphine!

  Also I really think you should be told about the volume of blood you will lose as a period! The hospital kept telling me to look out for blood clots when I went to the toilet and I was home a day when I was just standing talking on the phone when a massive blood clot fell out of me into my underwear! I panicked and rang my Doctor and they checked me out but I was told it was normal! I hadn't been told that! Also for getting in and out of bed you really need a pillow to hold up against your tummy and its also helpful for coughing or laughing!

- Having had one elective emergency section with no labour and having given birth naturally at full term, I would chose natural birth 10 times over to avoid a c-section. There is no comparison. Natural births can go as wrong as well, we know that, but for sure there is a difference in bonding and the release of hormones etc. and the recovery time; the pain. I didn't have a baby to lift as she was in ICU but I had to go to the ICU everyday and how else was I going to do it only by driving—after 2 weeks of having others pick me up and drop me off. For me it robbed me of everything a first timer thought it would be about but then again any version of a harrowing birth can rob you of all the things you thought it would be. For any first timer reading this and worrying... don't. I am still happy and healthy and so is my daughter 7 years on. We do get over it!

- I have had two sections one emergency and one elective. The emergency section was after a long labour where I was fully dilated and pushing but my son was stuck as he was in a posterior position so I had to have an emergency section as he was in distress. There were only two things that upset me: First, I am very claustrophobic and the drapes were far too close to my face and when I tried to explain it to the theatre staff they thought I was panicking and kept shushing me! I was furious about that but realise their prerogative was to get the baby out!
Secondly, they whipped him away and I didn't get to even look at him when he came out—he needed suction and oxygen and took what seemed like an age to cry! It was all very frightening and for weeks I kept looking at him wondering was he really my baby as I hadn't seen him when he came out—it made it more difficult to bond. My daughter was born by elective section 3 weeks ago and it was a lovely positive experience! The staff were so nice chatting away to me and distracting me when the epidural was going in. I even got to watch the whole operation on a TV screen which I didn't think I'd want to look at but I ended up telling my husband to move his head out of the way! When they lifted her out they put her straight onto my chest for a kiss and a cuddle and then she was cleaned up! I found no difficulty bonding this time and absolutely knew she was mine! The

surgeon removed my previous section scar which had become infected twice and was like a raised red welt on my tummy and I now have a lovely neat barely noticeable scar that healed very quickly and didn't get infected! When I was back on the ward there was a nursery nurse who offered to take her at night for a couple of hours—I was reluctant the first night but was glad of the rest the second night! All in all the staff were absolutely wonderful and having such a positive experience this time helped me overcome my fear and post traumatic stress of my first experience.

- On my first pregnancy I was induced due to high blood pressure and protein in my urine and got to pushing for 75 minutes but ended up with an emergency section—I know in hindsight being an emergency that it was all rush rush rush but I now believe if someone had taken just 5 minutes to explain everything to me things may not have ended up as bad as they did. No one explained that although I would feel no pain I would feel them working on me, this completely and utterly freaked me out, I started shaking uncontrollably and simply couldn't stop, I started losing a lot of blood and ended up with a general anaesthetic. When I got pregnant again the delivery was an issue that I just couldn't think about. After a long talk with my consultant (and lots of tears on my part) we decided it was very likely I'd end up with a bigger baby and most likely another section (1st babs 9lb, 2nd babs 9lb 8oz). It was a completely different experience—everything was explained to me and everything done to keep me calm— if I started to feel panic I just had to call out and someone immediately was at my side just talk to me and calm me—I couldn't believe the difference in the experience—I was back on the ward with my baby in my arms in approx 2 hours, I don't even remember the first 24 hours of my eldest. I do know that part of the reason for a better experience 2nd time around was I'd been there before and I'm also aware that 1st was an emergency so maybe no time for me but the difference in taking the time to talk to me both before and during the procedure made a huge huge difference for me.

Deborah

- I found out the day before my due date that baby was breech and I would have to have a section. He's just turned six months and I'm still raw and struggling to come to terms with the experience. It's very hard to put into words the feelings that I had but I think the most overwhelming feeling was the lack of control. I just lay there unable to move while everyone around me carried on with what was just day to day routine to them but to me it was life changing and there was no real sense of that. I wish I had known what sensations to expect.

  That although you don't feel pain you are aware of the pulling and tugging to get baby out and this made me feel very sick. I wished I had known that the sharp pain I got in my shoulder during the surgery happens sometimes. If I had known it was trapped air I wouldn't have been so distracted by it. Also wish I had known it sometimes lasts for a few days afterward. I wish I had known that they clean you up down below afterwards. I was so uncomfortable with this. At least after a normal delivery you can get your dignity back once baby arrives. I wish I had known that you need help going for a shower the next day. I actually would have been fine, but they would not allow me to go alone. Thank God my partner was there to take me or it would have had to have been a nurse. I wish I had known that you have to wear those God awful socks that help your circulation even though they feel like they are strangling you. I wish I had known that you have to get an anti clot injection in your thigh twice a day. I wish I had known that the area around my scar would be numb for months after.

- For me I wish someone had told me that to plan in the event of the epidural or spinal didn't work, to tell your partner, not to let everyone know what you had until you came around from general anaesthetic, I found that everyone from family to work colleagues knew I had a son, and his weight, who he like etc, three whole hours before I did and I was the person who carried him for nine months—that was very distressing...

Veronica

- I had a section about 4 months ago. I was a week overdue so I was induced. My waters broke couple of hours later and soon went into labour. Found it very painful so got epidural. Great relief! I was in labour for over 11 hours, went to 9cm but failed to progress any further. Baby wasn't in distress or anything but the Doctor said they'd have to do a section because he wasn't coming out. I was delighted because they told me I was having a big baby, he was 9lb 10!. They prepped me for theatre, topped up epidural and off I went for the section. I was fine until I got into operating room and I got very nervous then. But everyone was so nice and explained everything they were doing. but then I heard someone say "oh this is after coming off"! It was one of the tubes, don't know if it was the epidural or what. But they started cutting and that was fine. Next thing I started feeling everything, and I mean everything. It wasn't that normal pulling feeling that people talk about, it was like they were pulling a football out of a hole the size of a grape. I could feel them pulling back the skin where they cut and rooting around. I was 9cm before I went in, so his head was well down and they had to pull him back up to get him out. I've never felt such pain in my life. I was screaming the place down and my knuckles were white as I held on to the operating table. They had to knock me out I was in such pain. Then I woke up as he was being born, thank god—I didn't want to miss that. But then I was screaming again asking if he's out why the hell am I feeling the same pain again. They explained they were taking out the placenta. That was as bad as taking him out! They knocked me out again, and when I woke this time, they told me they were just putting my womb back in!! Too much information for me, don't know whether they knocked me out here or if I passed out!! I felt very groggy and weepy after it, couldn't tell you what nurses were saying to me. But as bad as it was I would definitely go for a section next time, think I was just one of those horror stories you hear of! I would rather a section than get stitched or tearing, ouch! And the recovery was very fast, was up and about after a week, slowly mind you but up all the same. I didn't do housework for ages, I kept using the excuse of having had a 'major operation'!!

• I would like to tell you my story of my recent c-section. I had a planned caesarean section due to a medical condition which was planned for the 14th July. I had a beautiful baby boy weighing 8lbs 4oz. I was admitted on the Monday afternoon into admissions and went through the usual tests— blood pressure, blood tests and baby monitoring. We were there for about 2 1/2 hours and then got our room. It was nice to have the afternoon to ourselves. We had decided not to tell anyone when we were going in as they all would be ringing us asking for news and it would have wrecked our heads. Anyway my husband stayed with me until late that night and we both got an early night.

The minute he had left the nerves set in and I got so lonesome after him knowing this was the last night we would be on our own. Of course I didn't sleep much that night. I was up early as I was first down to theatre. My husband was in at 7.30am and I got my tablet to settle the acid in my stomach. We just sat on the bed waiting to be called by the nurse. We both were so nervous (this is our first!!) in less than an hour, we were going to be parents and we couldn't believe it had come so quick. We were then walked up to the theatre and I was given a liquid which settled any acid left in my stomach.

My husband wasn't allowed in while I was getting my spinal block and that was the one thing that I was so nervous and anxious about. When I walked in, everyone was doing their own jobs, so I ended up walking around the theatre on my own which helped me to calm down and see what was going on. Then the anaesthetist came over and introduced himself and his assistant and told me what they would be doing. So I got up on the side of the bed to prepare for the spinal block. The Midwife stood in front of me and I leaned over towards her, holding her hand. I bent over as they told me and they put in the local anaesthetic first which was fine and then the spinal, it was ok a bit uncomfortable but I did lots of deep breathing which I always find help me get through tough times. They then were pushing against a nerve and he had to stop and go up a bit higher in my back, at this stage I knew what to expect so it was ok.

He had told me that I had good posture as I wasn't bending over enough at times but that's thanks to Pilates. Straight away I felt like my toes were on fire and they moved me back on the bed. It was a strange experience not being able to feel your legs. My left leg started to fall off the bed but as hard as I thought I was trying I couldn't get it back up on the bed, so my consultant had to push it back up with her bum, I was laughing at her which help me to settle down. Then they sprayed water over my chest which I felt and they knew then it was ok to start. They put in a drip on my arm and took my blood pressure and she started. They then called my husband in and within 4 minutes our beautiful son was born.

I couldn't believe how quick it all was. I didn't feel a bit of her pulling him out or stitching me up, I suppose really when he was born I was so preoccupied with seeing him that I wasn't bothered what was going on below me. I did start to feel a bit nauseous but they gave me an injection to help. I was then brought out to the recovery room after about 20 minutes and I finally got to hold my son properly, we had asked to have skin to skin contact as I couldn't breastfeed either so he was put inside my gown and it was the most beautiful moment of my life. Oisín was fast asleep and I honestly thought this was the most special moment in our lives. We stayed here for another half hour and we were then brought back down to our room. I was very tired when I got back and I think I did doze off a bit and my husband gave our son his first bottle.

I was hooked up to fluids, morphine and had a catheter also. After about 2 hours I could start to wiggle my toes and at 4.30pm I was taken out of the bed by the nurse. I was a bit nervous as I had no underwear on, just 2 pads were put up against me and the mat was put on the bed underneath me. The nurse helped me out of the bed which was very painful, take your time and hold onto the nurse and just put out your legs one at a time and shift out your bum to the edge, that will help to get up. The nurse warned me that I may get a flood and not to be worried that this was normal and she just caught the bed sheet and pulled it up around me and we slowly walked into the bathroom. I did feel very weak but I got to the toilet and had a wash and put on my underwear and nightdress, straight away you feel so much better. I stayed in hospital for 4 days and I was allowed to go home on the Friday. I took my time every time I got up, don't rush around and take the morphine and painkillers that they offer. I would recommend using the green maternity pads that you get in the chemist, they are much better and are very cheap to buy.

Also if you can use toilet wipes as they are softer and cleans as well and this helps with any infection that may set in. Bring in little luxuries for yourself like Vitamin E spray as the hospital can be so warm and stuffy, lip balm and hand cream etc, just little things that will make you feel better. Also bring in some snacks as you will get peckish during the night and between meals during the day but also for your hubby too. The nurses will often take your baby at night time if they can which gives you a chance to get some sleep. Make the most of it.

All in all, I would go through it all again, I was so nervous beforehand but I just relaxed when I got into the theatre, looked around and spoke to all the staff in there and took plenty of deep breaths and just concentrated on what I was going to get out at the end. Take your time afterwards; watch yourself in what you do getting up and around. Do your pelvic floor exercises carefully and most of all enjoy your baby and being parents.

Martina

- I wish I'd known that you could be sick during the section—I threw up 3 times in the emergency section but when I asked for a kidney dish this time round just in case they gave me anti sickness meds and I was grand!

- I had two sections—one after a failed induction where I got to fully dilated and pushed for 90 minutes before the decision was made to move to a section. The only issue I would have with the section that time was that, due to the emergency of the situation, my partner was not fully informed what was going on. He waited in the hall while I was prepped and then was brought into the room to find me all hooked up to machines.

Obviously he knew I was having a section but he didn't have any idea what was going on while I was being prepped and was nervous enough about the whole thing. I did have a lot of shaking due to the drugs (this was not really explained to us as a reaction to the drugs but it wore off quickly) and I couldn't even look at the baby for an hour after I got to the recovery room. Once the shaking wore off I was fine and then I was able to feed the baby a little. I went back to my room at about 3am and the baby was kept for a few hours before being brought to me at the change of shift. I was lucky that I was not in much pain afterwards and got feeling back quickly but I had lost a bit of blood and so was fairly wiped out. The second section was elective—the labour did not start naturally and induction is not really an option. This was really straight forward: I went in expecting a similar experience but it was totally more relaxed with very few drugs in the operation and the whole thing was done in 2 hours.

I would say that the Midwives were great about helping out when I called them and that would be the key advice—they are not going to hang around your room looking to see if they can help out so it is up to you to call them to get help. I found that the staff where I had both my sections were more than willing to help. I had a private room in both instances and I think that the lack of company increased my sense of isolation when I had my first child. I didn't have a clue about what I was doing and he was a really hungry baby which meant that he slept little and I was constantly in demand. Other than the first night, I had him every night and it was tough going really. I think in hindsight I should have asked for more help but if the ward is busy it is difficult for the nurses to take the child for the full night. With the second child the Midwives took her for me for the first two nights and that was great. I was breastfeeding but they gave her a bottle at night and let me sleep. I didn't have any issue with bonding even though both babies went to recovery in an incubator before I ever held them. I hate when I see people saying that there are differences with bonding and hormones etc when you have a section. That is a generalisation that can have a very negative effect on those that are required to have sections every time they give birth. I don't think that I have missed anything by giving birth by section rather than having labour. I would most likely have been induced for both births and what I experienced of that was far worse than any section. To force the body to create contractions when it clearly is not interested in doing this can be just as traumatic for the mother—in my case I freely admit that I would have been very nervous having an induction in the second labour. Some things I would tell some one else having a section:

They put in a lot of drugs when it is an emergency section. I had a Doctor putting drugs in constantly once I was on the table. The shakes can happen in response to the drugs. Ask for help after your surgery. Drugs are up to you but I would accept whatever they suggest as you would after any major surgery. Go to the physio classes as there is good advice there. Don't get too caught up in how your baby was delivered. Just be glad that everything ended well and enjoy your child.

- Sounds very silly—had two sections, 1 emergency and 1 planned. Wish I had known that I would still feel the sensation of everything. Did not like the feel or sounds of the Doctor poking his hands around in side of me!

- To be honest I had a very good experience, I had an emergency section on the Thursday after having been induced on the Tuesday I was only 1cm after all that time my Doctor asked me if it was ok to do a c section and I agreed she gave me a quick scan and realised that my baby was tangled in the cord which was around her neck they started moving very fast then but it was all explained to me as we went along. My husband was very nervous but the staff were excellent they really reassured him while they were doing the operation a Midwife kept us up to date with what was happening. When she came out the Doctor showed her to us from a distance very quickly but just told us she needed help. Yes I would have loved to hold her straight away but her health and safety were more important I knew they would look after her, after the paediatricians looked at her I was allowed hold her for a few minutes before she was taken to neo natal and my husband went with her. The nurses down there were outstanding they took my mobile number and rang me to update me on her she was born at 1.17am and about 9am I was able to get up and have a shower with the help of a Midwife then she brought me down in a wheelchair and I spent the day with my baby. I got that shoulder pain but Solpadol helped with it. Coughing and laughing was very hard but I found the quicker I got up

44

and gently moved about it was easier to recover I'm not talking about doing a ten mile walk but taking it easy not just staying in bed. It was uncomfortable for about two to three weeks oh and if if the weather is cold remember to put extra layers by your scar it can be sensitive. Another thing don't try wear jeans stick to soft clothes.

- I had an emergency c-section due to foetal distress almost six weeks ago. To cut a long story short, labour wasn't progressing initially, baby's heart rate kept dropping, four foetal blood samples were taken from my poor son's head, I was given oxytocin and started to over-contract (thank GOD I'd had the epidural before that started), consultant arrived in and discovered that I had gone from 2-9 cm in an hour but that the baby had meconium grade 3 and he felt we couldn't wait the extra 2-3 hours it would have taken to deliver vaginally. 20 mins later my baby was out but was taken to special care because of the meconium. I second the other Mums who said that they found it quite traumatic—I thought it was just me.

In retrospect I think I went into shock a day or two after my son was born. Initially I was just so elated that I had had a baby (plus I think the morphine helped!) that the section didn't really affect me (apart from physically) but around day 3 I decided to walk down the hall to stretch my legs and when I got to the end of the ward discovered it was right beside the delivery suites and I just started to shake uncontrollably. I then spent about a week obsessing about the delivery—trying to piece it all together (it seemed to pass in a bit of a haze at the time), trying to come to terms with how it had happened, worrying whether everything had been done right and whether I should have insisted that my consultant came in sooner, feeling very upset that my child had been distressed and I hadn't really been thinking about him. In short, I feel the emotional impact of the section was absolutely huge. It may be that I was having baby blues and because I had a section I had more to focus on, but I think the impact of emergency sections is completely underplayed.

What I wish I'd known before:

Why didn't I seriously consider it? I had a near 'perfect' pregnancy—wasn't sick at all, blood pressure and urine absolutely normal at every hospital visit and in retrospect I think I was convinced that I was going to have a normal birth—the baby being distressed did not even occur to me as a possibility, which I felt hugely guilty about later. Even though I had devoured every pregnancy book going I don't think I had really contemplated it at all I found the whole medical staff's attitude to the section frustrating. Their words and actions seemed to conflict all the time—everyone kept saying 'you have had major surgery' yet all their actions suggested that a section is a routine and minor procedure. I did not have one person tell me how to care for my wound properly, or what to look out for in terms of it not healing correctly. The result was that I developed a nasty infection in my wound after 10 days which required antibiotics to clear and nearly put paid to breastfeeding my baby, as I couldn't lift him just as he was going through a growth-spurt. When I went back to the hospital to get it treated I was asked 'Did I not notice any redness or pain' and my answer was 'yes, of course I did, but I've just had my insides split open so I EXPECTED to have pain; I just didn't know that this was 'different'. The emotional impact, as detailed above. That being said, six weeks on I am convinced that the section was 100% the right thing to do in the interests of my son's welfare, so I am in no way angry or annoyed that it happened, or wished it had been different. He was clearly distressed and had been for some time, so the most important thing was that he was born safely and there is no way I would have endangered him by waiting the extra 2-3 hours to have a normal birth.

▌ Our Experience of Caesarean Birth—Part I—Anonymous

When we found out we were pregnant we debated having a home birth. We hadn't done enough research or thought sufficiently about it when the time came to make a decision however. Having heard hugely positive reviews of a particular Midwife scheme, we figured it was the next best thing. We worked hard on trying to put ourselves (well me really) into the best place for a natural birth. Not simply as a route to avoid drugs, but also to ensure that both I and my baby achieved the healthiest and happiest birth we could. I did yoga, active birth classes, read all the natural childbirth books I could lay my hands—the usual stuff. Despite this, I could never shake a deeply ingrained fear of labour. I used to lie awake at night panicking at the thought of what was ahead of me. Despite the reputation of the Midwives, my fears were never addressed. When I tried to raise them at my 38 week appointment, my hospital file was marked "overly emotional". This was hugely upsetting and I felt completely unsupported and unprepared for labour. I was warned from early in the pregnancy that despite my small stature I appeared to be growing a very large baby. Two days after my due date, my waters broke spontaneously. Gradually over the next 12 or so hours, contractions started. I was scared at being at home alone with just my husband.

Despite knowing that staying at home as long as possible is recommended we headed into the hospital. Unfortunately we met a very unsympathetic Midwife who gave me a sweep without asking my consent or explaining what she was doing. The contractions became intense very soon afterwards. I spent hours trying every position I could but nothing seemed to relieve the strong back labour I was experiencing. At one point when I felt completely out of control the Midwife assigned to me told me to pull myself together. It was awful. From that point on, it got worse. Nothing seemed to ease the pain and the constant suggestion to accept pain relief undermined my attempts to get through the labour naturally. Late that evening, after a long and painful

24 hours, the Midwife told me I was "only" 2cm dilated. I felt deflated and exhausted.

All that hard work and insane pain for nothing? I burst into tears and asked for an epidural. The one thing I wanted to avoid. I knew it meant succumbing to a series of interventions or assistance. But I was so tired and I simply couldn't cope with the pain. The epidural only worked on one side unfortunately. And what I didn't know was that I had been given oxytocin without my consent so I could feel the full force of artificially induced contractions on one side. It was agony. I clearly remember screaming in pain. I was completely panicked—the wait for the next contraction was almost as unbearable as the actual contraction. I finally hit the magic 10cm and was told I "could push now". But I couldn't feel anything. I had to lie back despite my body aching to sit up. It was impossible. There was no way my body could force such a large baby out when I was in such an unnatural position. They started mentioning sections, operating theatres and surgeons. It all happened so quickly. Next thing I knew, my husband was gone and I was alone in a room full of gowned and masked strangers.

They attempted a ventouse and then a forceps delivery but there was no budging my big baby. I begged to be allowed to push for longer but the angle of the operating table was such that all I achieved was slipping off. When my husband was finally allowed in, we were both in tears. I was unceremoniously sliced open and my precious baby was whisked away from me without a word. I could hear people in the corner of the room exclaiming at how big he was but I hadn't even seen him. The fact that the first people he saw was not his father and I, the fact that the first hands to hold him were not loving hands breaks my heart and still brings me to tears nearly 3 years later. I didn't get to touch him, to hold him, to love him for nearly 5 hours. As for the golden 30 minutes of breastfeeding, not a chance. He was sent alone, screaming, to a crowded nursery while I lay in agony in a cold and sterile recovery room with a nurse who couldn't explain where my baby was or why I couldn't be near him. Hardly the best first hours of life.

When we were finally united, he was washed and dressed. He could have been anyone's baby. I begged for help feeding him but received none. I was doped up with morphine and my poor baby was too probably. The first few days were a disaster. At every turn I was told he was too big a baby and he needed formula. I was exhausted and my poor son was slowly starving.

It's no wonder I found it difficult to bond with him. Breast feeding was next to impossible, despite me paying for professional help. (I'm still waiting for the lactation consultant from the hospital to call!). I felt like a failure. I had failed to bring my precious baby into the world the right way and now I was failing to feed him. I simply could not cope with the range of emotions I was feeling over his birth. I felt like something was missing—I still needed to push him through me, to finish the cycle or complete the circle. I was at a loss. I don't know why my baby's birth happened the way it did. I don't believe it was simply because he was a large baby. I believe the maternity system failed me— failed to prepare me and failed to support me when it came to crunch time. I will never forgive the hospital, the Midwives and the experience for depriving my son and I of a normal birth. It has taken years for me to heal emotionally.

I will always carry the scars, and not just the horrible one across my abdomen. I still feel terrible pain when I think about my son's birth, but I'm lucky that he is such an incredibly beautiful child and it is exceptionally easy to love him. Is it any wonder I planned a homebirth when I got pregnant the second time? Deciding to have a homebirth was one of the best decisions I ever made. The minute the Midwife walked into our home and spoke to my husband, son and I, I knew we had made the right decision. We trusted her completely. I knew we were in safe hands (literally and figuratively).

■ Part II

The pregnancy was uneventful. I hated my previous pregnancy but this was different. I looked forward to the Midwife's visits. It was a chance to ask questions at my own pace, to voice my worries, to simply relish being pregnant. But more than anything else, every visit compounded my belief that we had made the right decision. I was looking forward to labour, something, after my first son's birth, I never in a million years though I would be able to say. My Midwife instilled such confidence in me—birth is a normal natural event, something to be enjoyed and celebrated. Despite my Midwife having seen hundreds of birth, she still radiated an excitement about the wonder and miracle of birth. It was an absolute joy being around her. She seemed unfazed by my previous Caesarean section and simply made a birth plan to accommodate it.

As I was hoping for a VBAC at home, there was lots of irritating red tape to get through and several times throughout the pregnancy we thought our home birth dreams were over. It was a stress we could have done without. But our belief and faith in our Midwife never wavered, nor did her commitment to me and my baby.

The hospital I had registered with for scans and bloods were less than helpful. In fact one consultant obstetrician actively sought to bully, intimidate and scare me. It didn't work, if anything it reaffirmed our belief that home was where our son should be born.

I knew I would go into labour early. I knew the baby was big and wanted out, sooner rather than later. A week of intense warm ups pushed my "gentle birth" techniques to the test.

The day he was born, I was tired after yet another night of pacing the floor with contractions. I had just decided to have an early night when my waters broke. I phoned my Midwife. My husband was upstairs putting our son to bed and I was flooding the downstairs. I could see my bump dramatically shrinking with the volume of liquid I was loosing. My sister—who was to look after our older son was out of contact. Quite quickly the contractions started. They were incredibly strong and frequent. I started to panic, I barely had time to breath between contractions and I was all alone.

By the time my Midwife arrived—less than 10 minutes after I had called—I was in full labour. A quick check showed me to be 5cm and ready to go. Everything was happening so fast I wasn't registering anything. I got into the pool and breathed through strong contraction after strong contraction. My Midwife asked if I wanted to transfer for pain relief and I very definitively declined. It was hard but there was no way I was not going to experience this. Just before transition I had time to sit back in the pool for a much needed breather. It was the most unusual, surreal experience, I was in incredible pain yet I clearly remember laughing that a friend had predicted that this labour would be fast and furious. I remember cursing her accuracy. Baby was progressing well and I started pushing. He was happy throughout.

The Midwife got me to change position. Then I heard her say "we need to go". I knew that transfer to hospital meant another caesarean section. I was vaguely aware of her calling for an ambulance and calling for my sister to get my bag together but I was not in their realm. The paramedics tried to get me into the ambulance as I struggled through expulsive contractions. I remember hunkering down at my front gate as yet another urge to push engulfed me and noticing my neighbours feet as he walked by. What a sight he must have seen. I was in another world though, lost in my body and the experience. I knew what was happening but was completely unable to interact with the drama unfolding around me. It was just me and my little one.

Unfortunately our arrival at the hospital was less than welcomed. The consultant who we had previously had difficulties with was on call. She seemed almost gleeful that her dire predictions had come true. She accused me of not trying hard enough, of making it more difficult for myself and warned me that I would regret making such a poor effort. She ignored my Midwife's explanation that I had been pushing for nearly two hours and that baby's progress was obstructed. She forced me to undergo a rough examination and shouted at me when I complained. She ignored my repeated requests for a surgical delivery. It was horrendous. The contractions, which had been hard but manageable in the pool at home were now completely overwhelming. I was exhausted, scared and in unbearable pain. My Midwife had warned us that I may have to fight for a section (the irony was not lost on me) so my husband intervened and demanded action. Only when we threatened to take the matter to her superior did she relent and start the process for theatre.

While operating she maintained a constant dialogue with all but me. My son was born, healthy and roaring with gusto. Knowing the process, I demanded immediate contact and a short recovery separation period. My request for the placenta was sarcastically criticised and denied. How I wished I had the energy to fight more.

Despite the awfulness of the ending I was euphoric. I had my beautiful baby in my arms and he nursed enthusiastically. The experience of labouring in the pool was still strong and fresh in my mind and I felt like I had birthed my son. I sat awake all night gazing at him and marvelling at the wonder of it all.

I couldn't believe the Doctor on call the next morning was the same consultant. Did she ever go home? On day two after yet another experience of her rudeness, lack of compassion and downright ignorance I demanded to see another Doctor.

Thankfully this blot has not affected my joy in my son's birth. He is a glorious creature and my heart swells with love when I look at him. No amount of sleepless nights can dim my absolute delight in his being. And that is in no small way attributable to his homebirth journey into the world and the care, support and love we received from our Midwife.

- Some parts of this story may be very difficult to read particularly for Mums to be. However our story is not typical of the majority of births and therefore no one should ever feel that this may happen to them and at the end of it all I have a beautiful healthy baby, who was brought into the world safely. I am writing this as I feel it is important to share all stories. I wish mine had been a successful and good hypno story as I had worked hard before the birth for this however the important thing is that my baby is beautiful, healthy and happy.

During my pregnancy I was completely sure and positive that I would have a successful hypno birth. Ever since I was young I imagined that I would have a good labour, I imagined having an active labour, walking on the beach near home before going into the hospital. I imagined arriving in hospital and already being several centimetres dilated. During the pregnancy I did yoga, reflexology and used Raspberry leaf tea towards the end and we also did perineal massage. I envisioned enjoying my labour and recovering well afterwards. I wrote a very clear birth plan, stating that I wanted minimal interventions i.e. none of the "otomies" episiotomy, amniotomy and I preferred to labour without an epidural or other drugs. I wanted to remain active in the labour to ensure a shorter second phase. However all of this preparation helped mentally for what was to be the reality of my labour but did not help physically.

Saturday 20th 5 am: Got up went to loo and before I even got there felt a trickle of fluid thought hmm interesting and wondered if my waters were breaking. I put a pad on and an hour later there was very little on it so dismissed it and assumed it was not my waters. Then an hour later had lots of big blobby mucus and tiny bit of pink so thought it was the mucus plug. This continued for the day.

Sat evening 8 pm started to get menstrual cramps, nothing unusual there, but suddenly they started forming a pattern and feeling stronger until about 1am more pink mucus and at this stage the cramps were every 5-7mins and had been for an hour. We decided it was time to go to the hospital and off we went the contractions were then coming every 3—5 mins by the time we got there and all I had learned in yoga and hypnobirthing kicked in even stronger and I really managed them. We were admitted and I had my first internal by 2 am and sadly I wasn't dilated at all however she said the cervix was effaced and baby was well down and things were happening so no need to go home as it was all definitely kicking off, at this internal the membranes were deemed to be intact.

I was then transferred to a ward and got a bed but spent the rest of the night with contractions still coming every 3-5mins and lasting up to 60 seconds, walking, squatting using the ball etc etc by 6 am I had had 2 other internals and this is when they realised my waters had gone. Hubby was sent away to rest as it was felt it would be a while before I started to dilate. I was so fed up that despite at this stage 10 hours of regular contractions I wasn't dilating at all but the staff weren't worried so I continued with it. Hubby didn't want to go home so instead he slept in the car and got a good five hours sleep. I continued to walk and squat through the contractions as had been advised to help with dilation.

Sunday 11am another internal and the team were beginning to worry that despite the intensity and regularity of the contractions I still wasn't dilating so the decided to "induce" me

I didn't know whether to laugh or cry at the irony of being induced when I had been having contractions for 15 hours already. Anyway they moved us back to delivery and started me on oxytocin and a monitor for babies heart and my contractions. So sadly I was confined to bed at this stage which made the contractions much more difficult however I was determined that at least I would have a better second stage and faster second stage so continued without the epidural for another four hours. I continued with my yoga, hypnobirthing and calming techniques and using lovely music.

We had a lovely room and my husband was super talking me through it as was our assigned Midwife. However the oxytocin was really doing its job and I was having 8 contractions every 15 mins they had to keep reducing the levels and switching it off as they said that anymore than 7 is nearly dangerous... The contractions often didn't even have a break between them so hubby and I had a serious chat about the epidural. My reasons for not having it were already fading as it had been because I wanted to have an active labour and now with the oxytocin this was not possible as I had to be on the bed. No one had any idea how long more this was gonna go on because four hours in I STILL HADN'T DILATED so I took the epidural. The staff were brilliant because despite the fact that already I had had some interventions they continued to follow my birth plan as much as possible and discussed all the merits etc of everything being suggested.

Anyway eventually 6 hours after the oxytocin I was 1 cm dilated. I finally begin to feel my body was not as useless as I thought. However it took 9 hours in total to get to eight cm dilated and this lasted another 3 hours at about 9pm I became violently ill but was only vomiting bile as I hadn't eaten since about 7pm on Saturday evening, and then I got excruciating pain in my groin so the anaesthetist was called again. We believed that the vomiting were things really beginning to happen and got very excited. However, by midnight on Sunday it was decided I couldn't continue, I'd had nearly twelve hours of oxytocin and had been at 8cm for four hours and the Doctor was concerned during this internal that baby was face up with a tilted head and did not think I could deliver naturally. So all systems became go and a c section was happening, I was crushed after all we'd been through, I would now be more incapacitated, pumped with drugs, bed bound, longer in hospital etc but the staff were brilliant, telling me how well I had done and how soon I would have babs.

WARNING—THIS IS THE SCARY BIT. The section began. Hubby was there, the team were ready, I was numb, but a few minutes into the surgery I started to sense a burning sensation on my left side I said it to the anaesthetist and he began trying to deal with it but the surgery was beginning to get complicated and they were struggling to get the baby out as he was so far down my pelvis and because the position is head was in etc so I began to get freaked out with all the tugging and pulling and this burning sensation and I started to loose consciousness, then hubby was asked to leave. Anyway we got through it and my husband was brought back in as they got baby out and when I saw this head of black hair I bawled and the pain suddenly wasn't as noticeable. Baby was absolutely fine despite everything although initially they thought they had broken his shoulder trying to get him out— they hadn't and he was fine. I was sent to recovery where it took an hour to get the pain under control and the anaesthetist was so apologetic about the pain I'd felt during the surgery and good to me as I was so all over the place.

I was back on the ward with my baby boy to my breast by 4.30 am and he has been thriving every since. I am still quite slow and uncomfortable but hoping this will soon go.
Emotionally though I feel very raw. I am so disappointed that I was unable to deliver naturally and I am so upset that I am slow and uncomfortable and physically unfit at a time when I

need to be at my best for the sake of my baby. I feel embarrassed when walking in public and want to tell everyone my story. The reality is there is no one to talk to after an emergency c section to help you understand your feelings and emotions. We brought our son to the Doctor for his two week check up and I thought I would be seen as well to ensure I was ok but the Doctor said it was just for the baby. I read everything I could to understand the recovery process better and what is normal and what is not as I got very little information about this in the hospital, but despite this I missed an infection which developed around five weeks post op, even for this I had to attend a GP as the hospital does not do follow up.

I am beginning to recover emotionally now but I am still so worried should I decide to have another baby, I really would want to have a natural delivery but I don't know what supports there are for this.

I feel in many ways traumatised by the whole experience and I feel I lost my dream birth and the bond that a natural birth creates for you and your baby and I feel disappointed in my body. Physically I do feel better but no where near pre pregnancy strength and fitness and I have no idea when or if I ever will. The hospital does offer exercise classes and advice from physiotherapists so now that I am six weeks post op I am going to attend these and hopefully get some support with the physical recovery.

So there you have it, long and difficult reading but as I say I have a beautiful boy.

▌ The Birth Story from Dad's point of view

When the Midwife suggested that my wife might need a section I was very disappointed for her. Not only had we been in the hospital for over 30 hours, with my wife having natural contractions, but then she was put on oxytocin and an antibiotic drip and for 12 hours had been confined to bed everything she had not wanted and had prepared so hard to avoid. I wasn't sure how she would feel about the section as I knew she really had not wanted this. However part of me was relieved as at that point I just wanted our baby delivered and the labour over for both him and my wife.

The Midwife explained what would happen and I was going to be allowed into the theatre with my wife. When I sat down beside my wife in the operating theatre I was determined to stay focused on her and not pay any attention to what the Doctors where doing. I had been warned to be careful not to touch or knock against anything but I was able to touch my wife's shoulder. I am not sure she was aware of this but it comforted me as the operating theatre was a little daunting, there were lots of people all doing different things and no one was really paying me any attention.

The surgery started as soon as I arrived and I just concentrated on the thought I would soon be seeing my son after waiting almost two days of labour (and nine months !) to meet him. While the surgery began the anaesthetist was asking my wife if she could feel anything and she kept repeating over and over that she could feel burning, she seemed to be concentrating very hard on getting through the surgery and I am not sure she was really describing how uncomfortable or painful the surgery was becoming. Each time my wife described the burning sensation the anaesthetist looked at another man who seemed to be supervising and when this person nodded they seemed to top my wife up with more drugs. I am not sure what they were giving her but she seemed to be losing the battle at this stage and began to drift into unconsciousness.

At this point I was asked to leave the room, I was waiting in a room nearby for about ten minutes and no one was telling me what was going on, I wondered if I was going to loose either my wife or my son. I was worried but I pushed it to the back of mind and let my mind continue to concentrate on the fact that I was going to meet my son very soon and then the three of us would be together. If I had been ten years younger than my 37 years I think I would have fallen to pieces at this stage. I think that life experience gave me the strength to get through these ten minutes by toughening me up. I decided not to ask anyone any questions about what was happening as I wanted them to just concentrate on my wife and son.

Finally I was let back into the room, my wife seemed a little out of it but was awake again and able to talk to me a little. Our son was finally free from the birth canal and in the world and as he was lifted away from my wife we could see his head of black hair, I was a little stunned that he was finally here and he was safe and saw my wife turn to me with tears in her eyes. There were a few minutes of fussing over the baby to make sure he was ok as it had been a difficult delivery and there was some concern that his shoulder was fractured from all the tugging to get him here. A day or so later it was confirmed for definite that his shoulder was fine but we were fairly certain that night that he was ok.

I spent the next two hours on my own with the little man and could not wait for my wife to join us as I knew how much she had wanted to put the baby to her breast as soon as possible after his birth and I knew this two hour separation would be killing her and this broke my heart.

Finally at 4am all three of us were together again and our son was in his mothers arms feeding from her breasts, the way it was meant to be.

The c section experience was traumatic and upsetting and the recovery has been tough for my wife, but our son was delivered successfully after becoming firmly wedged in the birth canal and therefore the surgery was necessary. My wife has found the recovery period slow and difficult but the remaining external scar is so neat it seems testament to me of a surgery well done.

- I was feeling very anxious for an unknown reason in the run up to my due date which was 4th August. I knew in my heart of hearts that I would not see that due date, I was preparing for week 39. As it turned out, I gave birth via emergency caesarean section two weeks and one day early. It was late on Sunday night and I had been asleep. My mobile woke me. It was a phone call from my mother in law to say that my sister in law had given birth two hours previously to her first baby. I remember hanging up the phone and smiling in the dark, delighted for the new parents and thinking how excited they must be feeling. I was still smiling on my way to the bathroom and wondering should I go downstairs to inform Mister Husband that he was an uncle or wait till he came up to bed. It was our seventh wedding anniversary and he was enjoying a drink, albeit solitary, downstairs. I didn't get a chance to decide. I finished my wee and immediately there was an audible "pop" followed by a steady release of fluid. I was delighted with myself. There go my waters I thought, fancy that. What are the chances of two first cousins being born within hours of each other? And two boys as well. This is going to be great! But hold on, surely I should be finished leaking at this stage. I knew I was retaining a lot of water but this was ridiculous. Then it stopped and I prepared to stand up. It started again and this time I felt a large clot pass. Straight away I knew this wasn't right. My waters hadn't gone. I was bleeding. And heavily. I banged on the floor with my foot as hard as I could and heard Mister Husband run upstairs. "Michelle and Ger have a baby boy," I told him, "All's well. Don't panic but I'm bleeding." "Shit, Gwen. I've been drinking." I can still recall being as cool as a cucumber as I issued instructions for the phone. I was going to ring my sister who would come down to stay with our sleeping sons and Mister Husband was to ring his father for a lift to the hospital. As soon as my sister was on the way, I called the hospital and explained briefly what was happening to me. I was told I could not wait the twenty minutes for my sister to arrive at our house and then travel another 40 minutes to the hospital. I was haemorrhaging and needed to travel to the hospital via ambulance and Mister Husband could follow me.

I grabbed my dressing gown, stuck three maternity pads in my pants, Mister Husband grabbed my hospital bag and within 10 minutes, the ambulance was outside our front door. I could still feel the blood and knew from a previous haemorrhage that I could pass out. I concentrated on my breathing as the lovely paramedic helped me into the ambulance, and took my details. I could feel the beginnings of very mild cramps and despite the air of urgency, I was excited. I was going to meet my baby! We arrived at the hospital and I was put on a monitor straight away. When Mister Husband arrived we asked our questions. The bleeding wasn't stopping and there was a strong possibility that I would give birth via caesarean section. It came as a shock as I had had two previous normal births and naturally enough, never entertained for a second that this would not be the case again. My head was still dealing with all of this new information but I managed to convey that it was of the utmost importance, both to me and Mister Husband, that skin to skin contact should be immediate after delivery and breastfeeding should be initiated as soon as possible.

We were reassured that this would be the case in any event. I couldn't explain it, but I felt a strong need to repeat my wishes and stress that they be carried out. In the event, of course, that I was going to be sectioned. This still had not been clarified. After a short while, another Doctor came in, removed the phone from the wall and informed theatre that they were to prepare for an emergency section. Mine. Then she looked at the Midwife that had been taking care of me, and asked her for consent forms. This was really happening. I had to ask them to slow down.

Everything was moving so quickly and it all seemed to be taken out of my hands. One minute I was being told that there was a possibility of a section and the next; I was shown the baby's trace and told how he was not doing well. There was talk of an epidural and how Mister Husband would be coming into theatre with me.

I believe less than hour had passed at this stage. Obviously the severity of the situation dictated that a section was the only way to go and I signed the consent form, gave it a kiss, and handed it over. At least, I thought, I would be awake and get to hold my baby immediately.

On the way to theatre however, I was not looking forward to the inevitable sensation of a surgeons hands pulling and tugging my baby out of my belly and into the world. Theatre is always a scary place. It's so sterile, shiny and bright. And all those masked faces with smiley eyes. The fact that you are lying on your back, in an extremely vulnerable position, does not help matters either. Still though, me being me, I decided to help them and obligingly started to roll over, all the better for them to stab me in the back with their epidural needle. I just wanted it over and to have my baby in my arms.

Suddenly the goal posts started to move again and this was before any drugs had been administered so it wasn't blurry vision. There was no need for me to roll over apparently as I was going to have a general anaesthetic. My arm was being tightly secured in a tourniquet and the back of my hand smartly rapped as a voice without a body sternly informed me that my baby was in danger and had to be delivered immediately. There was no time to administer an epidural and then wait up to twenty minutes to see if it would work. Did I understand? This was an emergency.

For the first time since I had been wheeled through the hospital doors, I heard the words "placental abruption." It would be two days later before I heard them again, followed by two more, "medical catastrophe." Fuuuuccccckkkk!! What could I do? Who was going to tell Mister Husband, who was waiting patiently outside the door, that he would not now be allowed into theatre? I was nodding my head whilst clutching a gas mask as the same voice without a body was telling me to inhale deeply, that I would feel someone pressing on my throat, and just to relax. Relax now. Relax. Relaaaaaaxxxx................ "Gwen? Gwen?" I opened my eyes five seconds later to see a tiny bundle dressed in white in Mister Husband's arms.

Mister Husband was calling my name and handing our son to me for a kiss. I can remember smiling like an idiot, kissing both Mister Husband and the baby (our third boy!!!!) asking Mister Husband "how lucky are we?" and then closing my eyes again. Oh, it was not five seconds later. It was an hour and a half. More on this later. Shortly afterwards. The next few recollections may not be in sequence. I apologise. Bear with me. There is nothing worse than that "I'm going to throw up" feeling. Except when you are on the flat of your back, unable to move, catheter in place and looking up at a stern faced nurse preparing a syringe. I was starting to retch. "I'm going to be sick. Can you help me up?" I asked. "In a minute." Stern Face continued with her syringe. I was visualising vomit on my face and in my hair. "Can you help me up? Please?" I was starting to panic. Again I was told, in a firmer tone of voice, "In a minute." I didn't have a minute. "Can you help me up, please?" This time I was attempting to sit up myself. "When I'm ready."

Unbelievably Stern face was still playing with her needle. But thankfully, she put it down to help me up. I learned the next day that Mister Husband had an incident with the same nurse. Once our son was safely delivered, approximately ten minutes after I disappeared behind those theatre doors, Mister Husband was called in. He was present all the while our baby was being checked over by a paediatrician who pronounced him hale and hearty. He shook Mister Husbands hand and left the room. Mister Husband was then told that I would be a further thirty minutes or so and he was asked to take a seat in the parenting room to wait. Someone would be out to him shortly.

After an hour when people were coming and going, but nowhere near him, he decided to ask about me. He met Stern Face who told him she didn't know and had no way of contacting theatre, before continuing on her way. At this stage he was beside himself. The thirty minutes had stretched into an hour and a half. After another search for a nurse and some reassurance, he was finally told that I would be down in five minutes. This is indeed what happened.

Later on that same night, Stern Face put pressure on Mister Husband to have our son bottle fed. He explained to her how important breastfeeding is to me and that I have previously fed two other children for 15 months each. It was my wish that this baby be breastfed only and unless there was a medical emergency, this was to remain the case. It was to be my decision and my decision only.

Shortly afterwards again. Trying to breastfeed. If this sounds like I was out of it, it's because I was. Both of us were. It's like a dream to me that I managed to crawl, or maybe I was pulled, into a semi sitting position, to offer my breast to our son. He half heartedly took it but it seemed, like me, all he wanted to do was sleep. I wish I had been warned about the unbelievable tiredness that would come afterwards. Shortly afterwards yet again. Tea and toast time. Manna. Absolute manna. Please sir? Can I have some more? Yet even later. It was time to decide what to do. The baby was still too sleepy to feed and I agreed for him to be cup fed in the nursery. Those two nurses were fantastic. They were understanding and supportive. He took one ounce. It was also time for Mister

Husband to go home and tell the big brothers that their little brother had arrived. We decided to call him Liam.

The next day—Monday was a wash out. Immediately on waking up, I thought of my two boys at home and I began to cry. I was missing them already. There was a morphine drip in the back of my hand for my convenience which was a major contributing factor to the incredible tiredness I was feeling. I even found it hard to talk. I refused food. I watched, completely redundant, as Mister Husband and the nurses changed Liam's nappy and lifted him in and out of the cot in order for me to feed him. He had to have another top up that day. If I felt like crap, he must have felt worse.

I wish someone had told me that Diphene and Ponstan were an alternative to morphine. In my case, a much better alternative. My catheter was removed that afternoon and I was helped out of bed. To say I felt like a ninety year old woman with severe arthritis, is an understatement. The sexy white support stockings did nothing for my self esteem either.
I told myself I bore a striking resemblance to Nicole in Home and Away but had more than a sneaking suspicion I was more like poor old Colleen when she goes to Bingo! I remember hobbling down the corridor clutching the arm of a nurse. I walked from my ward to the next ward and had to turn around. I was exhausted. Never before had I wanted a hot shower as much as I did that evening, but I knew it wasn't going to happen. I just was not up to it. Plus, it was time to get breastfeeding established. I had to call the Midwives when I wanted to feed Liam and although he still wasn't very interested, I was delighted to discover that it was indeed possible to feed sitting up.

The fact that I still had a nice round belly helped. I was able to prop him up on that and all the extra padding, protected my wound. After the first day, things began to get clearer. I was able to have my shower, but needed a chair to sit on for fear of becoming dizzy. One nurse told me not to do this alone but another led me into the bathroom and showed me where the alarm was if I needed it. I was left to my own devices after that.

Thankfully all my fears about breastfeeding post caesarean proved to be unfounded. Liam was feeding well once we got down to business. He was still sleepy but was actually feeding so I was happy and his nappies were an excellent indication that he was doing ok. And my milk came in at about the same time as it did on our second son, which was day three.

What I was not prepared for nor advised about was the havoc a section would wreak on my innards. Oh my god. I didn't have a bowel movement until day three and the night before I had to call the night staff and plead for some kind of relief. I knew what I was feeling was not "after pains" although I was experiencing these too. I was full of wind, gaseous, my tummy was so distended it was rock hard and feeding Liam that night was extremely difficult. It was like being pregnant with twins who were having a rave inside me. My stomach rocked and rolled, popped and gurgled and hissed until I was given a peppermint capsule. I was extremely sceptical as I swallowed it down but within ten minutes, I was releasing wind for Ireland. The relief was extreme.

The scar itself was not a problem. It was the maelstrom of emotions after the operation that took me by surprise. Nobody tells you about this. I hated the fact that other people had to look after my baby for the first couple of days until I was in a position to. I felt completely redundant. I was also ambushed by feelings of guilt over my other children being at home without their mother. I felt bereft and when I spoke to Mister Husband and the boys briefly each morning, I was in floods of tears afterwards. Tears because I missed them so much and although, I was the first thing they mentioned when they woke up, I was quickly forgotten as they went about their daily business. There was also, a very, very brief, scary moment that maybe this was not my baby sleeping peacefully in his cot at my bedside.

After all, I was unconscious when he made his dramatic entrance into the world. Too late, though, I had already bonded and no-one was going to take this child away from me, be he mine or someone else's. Mister Husband later reassured me that he was our flesh and blood.

If I needed further proof, I only had to read the many emails that were pouring in from family and friends proclaiming that he was the spit of our oldest child and announcing that Liam "has his Daddy's head on him." Another thing that I had heard about, and indeed, experienced the second time I gave birth were the fabled after pains everyone talked about. But these were different this time round. Much, much different. They were so sharp, so vicious they literally took my breath away.

It felt like there was a fist taking hold of my entrails, twisting hard and yanking downwards with great force, so much so that I was woken up at times with my fist stuffed in my mouth in an attempt to stifle a cry of pain.

Because I had haemorrhaged at home and lost more blood as a result of the operation, I was severely anaemic. A healthy haemoglobin count is 13. The day before I was discharged, I was 7.5. I was given an iron transfusion and warned that it would take up to five days to "kick in" but almost 5 weeks again before I would feel the full benefit of it.

In the days after being discharged from hospital, I parked myself on the couch in the front room out of sheer necessity. It was truly an enforced maternity leave. The after pains were still coming as brutally as before and I was slightly worried about my blood loss. Breastfeeding can mean that blood loss is minimal but I had stopped bleeding on the day I left the hospital. The PHN seemed to think I should be bleeding more and a Doctor advised that unless I was bleeding heavily, there was nothing to worry about. But I wasn't bleeding at all. There was also a huge build up of pressure in my pelvis. That, coupled with unbearable cramping at times, made me very fearful of an infection or another haemorrhage.

I was so glad to be getting out of hospital, I had neglected to ask what I should be aware of in the event of an infection. Typical of me, I thought of the questions to ask after the fact. Again, too late when I was home, it occurred to me that I hadn't received any aftercare advice either. I'd had various people at different times visit my bed side with leaflets on contraception, sterilising bottles, post natal depression, pelvic floor exercises and a how-to register your baby pamphlet. Bearing in mind that this was my third child, I considered myself to be fairly well versed in those matters already, but was pretty clueless in the caesarean section area. Which is exactly why five days after discharge, I went back to the hospital presenting with the above symptoms. Only to be told that they were all perfectly normal and to be expected. At the same time, I was put on a preventative course of antibiotics. Just to be on the safe side. I also replenished my supply of pain killers and Arnica.

Your stomach is your fulcrum, your prop, your support and it is only when you have what is considered to be major abdominal surgery, you discover just how often you use your stomach muscles. For everything. Coughing. Sneezing. Laughing. Even brushing your hair.

There is a six week recovery period post section and during this time you are advised not to drive, to refrain from hoovering and carrying out any heavy housework duties, anything, in fact, that requires a pushing and shoving movement. Carrying and lifting anything heavier than your baby is also very much advised against. What they don't tell you, is how you're supposed to carry on about your daily business without doing any of these things. How do you ignore your toddler who has his arms outstretched for a hug, to be lifted and comforted after he has had a tumble? What do you do when you're down to your last drop of milk and cannot drive to the shops for more. You can't even walk there and back.

Mister Husband and I are blessed with very supportive families who rallied round in our time of need. But I was still struck by how useless I felt. There were days, especially in the first couple of weeks, where I was literally unable to get out of bed. I suffered from sensory overload. I can recall one morning in particular. I had overdone it the day before by having a family breakfast in town and then pushing the buggy around for a half an hour. I was so exhausted the next morning, the sounds of our boys were like shards of glass piercing my brain. Mentally and physically over whelmed, I was reduced to tears.

One of the little luxuries I was looking forward to after I gave birth, was being able to roll over in my sleep without having to get out of the bed to do so. Three weeks after the section and I am no closer to this indulgence. I may not have to leave my bed in order to change sides but I am still cuddling up to a pillow to take the pressure off my scar and I still have to be careful getting in and out of the bed.

I realise I am only midway, at the very least, through the recovery process. It is not going to happen overnight. If some of what I've been reading of late is to be believed, the complete recovery time is a year at the most. I have read my fair share of pregnancy books and there is always a chapter concerning caesarean sections and a little piece at the beginning, imploring the reader not to skip. And they are all the same. They cover what it is like to have a section; the prep before theatre, what happens in theatre, tips for the mothers partner in theatre, tips for the mother in theatre, where to look, where not to look etc. etc.

I have yet to read a segment, any segment, on the recovery process. Nobody mentions how in the early days the scar can become red and raised, often with a burning sensation at one end. I never knew that numbness is very common. That this can last for a year or more, indeed some women never regain full sensitivity. Other women have complained of a breath taking pain in their shoulder. This is deferred pain from the section and not the beginnings of a heart attack. Another side effect is adhesions caused by scar tissue often needing more surgery to repair which in turn, can cause even more scar tissue.

There is also a one in one hundred chance that a section scar can rupture with a subsequent labour. The difficulties of going to the bathroom are ongoing. Haemorrhoids are a distressing pain in the proverbial. But the hardest reality of a section, I am finding, is the knock it can have on your confidence to bear another child. I am discovering that my family dynamic might have been changed forever. At this very moment in time I am nervous, scared even, at the thought of becoming pregnant again. I used to think that four or five children would be great. Our family was going to be finished by the time I was forty. But that has all changed now. It's something I'm not completely comfortable talking to Mister Husband about as he has already said that his family is not finished yet.

I can only hope that whatever decision we make will not have a detrimental effect on our relationship. For me, this last pregnancy was going to be a practice run for our fourth baby, one which I was hoping to have at home. The fact that I had an abruption of the placenta could render me an unsuitable candidate for a home birth.

Certainly the odds are slightly raised that I could haemorrhage again. All of these things, and more, have, at some stage, run through my head after the section and whereas I firmly believe that it is up to the individual to do their own research and have an arsenal of questions, at the same time, it would be so much nicer if a brief beforehand or immediately afterwards, was given.

- My name is Geraldine from Tallaght. My son just turned 1 the other day so its 12 months after my c-section, anyway I remember I was 5 days overdue and woke that morning to pains and assumed it was labour pain, decided to wait some hours to let the pain increase so I wouldn't have to be hanging around the hospital for hours until my son was born, anyway I did notice that day that my son hadn't really be kicking that day and they gave me a kick chart to keep track of his kicks as I was overdue so I rang up the Coombe and they said to come straight in, anyway went in and cant remember the name of it now but they strapped the strap around my waist to monitor baby's heart and see if I was actually having contractions, turned out I wasn't and the baby's heart rate was very slow so had to have an emergency c-section, as soon as I was told that it was like everything was rushed. One nurse pushing a form in front of my face to sign (I think if anything went wrong it was not their responsibility) and having to take off my jewellery and the toilet bag they attach so you don't wee while they are operating. I have to say it was very traumatic at the time especially as I had such a good pregnancy so certainly wasn't expecting things to happen that way when it came to the having baby part. I was crying and shaking so much I couldn't take out an earring. I remember there was one nurse who was so nice and trying to reassure me the whole time. Anyway I was brought into the theatre and I was asking for my partner to be brought in while they gave me the injection in my back to numb me up but they said he wasn't allowed in while they did that.

I felt they were so abrupt and rude, don't know if that's how they normally are, but the nurse who was nice to me held my hands as they gave me the morphine and did the normal preparation things.

If it wasn't for that nice nurse being there at the time I would have probably fainted with the shock of everything. Anyway after I was on the morphine obviously went relaxed, baby was born and didn't find out until 3 days later when my partner told me they had to re-suscitate the baby. In the end I had a healthy baby boy and was even let out on day four as I was healing so fast and they said baby has no bother with his heart thank god. The Doctor that delivered him came up to the ward two days after baby was delivered and asked if I knew why the baby had to be delivered by emergency c-section, I said yes because of his heart rate decreasing.

Anyway I did feel strange the next few days as this is my only child and I did feel robbed of giving birth to him. I'm ok with it all now and think ok the Doctors did save my baby and thank god for that but its still weird sometimes when I think back and wonder how did that happen, I went from a great pregnancy for the 9 months to bang—we are delivering your baby now.

Anyway that's my story and have just celebrated my baby boys 1st birthday and couldn't be happier he is in my life no matter what way he is born

- After a horrendous and traumatic "normal delivery" on no.1 I went on to have 2 elective sections under the care of my fantastic consultant. Both experiences were calm, painless and completely stress free. One thing to bear in mind is to check the hospitals policy on placing baby with you straight after. In the Coombe baby is placed skin to skin with you straight away in recovery and there's no waiting for an hour or so like other hospitals. I wish someone had told me that Granny knickers mean knickers up to you waist line and not just bigger ones!
I bought a size or so bigger on section 1 and they were brutal as they sat right on scar but on the second section those big sexy high waisted passion killers really did the job.

What someone did tell me was to get up and walk asap. On the first section the catheter was removed following morning and I walked about straight away. On my 2nd section I asked that catheter be removed that same evening and drank plenty of water to flush out bladder which worked a treat as I was up and about walking same day as op, my cannula (I think that's what the needle was called) came out same day as a result which was much more comfortable so if at all possible request removal of catheter as soon as possible.

I wish I'd known to that taking pain meds is just as important at home as it is in hospital as I let it lapse for a day thinking I was super human and suffered. Didn't make that mistake second time around!

- I had emergency caesarean on my daughter in 2006 after failed induction 11 days overdue. I wish I had known that:
  What you were told in that "15-20 minute slot" in the ante-natal class was a total gloss over of the truth of what would actually happen.
  You may not be re-united with your baby after the section until the full spinal block had worn off and that can take up to three hours.
  I would feel so devastated and such a failure at not being able to bring my baby into the world naturally. Something I still have trouble coming to terms with.
  I should have better prepared myself mentally for the possibility of a C-section.

The overwhelming jealousy I felt that my husband got to hold her, bathe her with the Midwives and dress her for the first time. Not that I begrudge that he got to do it but that I missed out on sharing that time with both of them.
The sheer agony of the operation on my body and that I couldn't move about properly for the first 3 days. That I would trip out so much on the painkillers and that they would cause so much sleep deprivation. That I could (and

did) have a urinary tract infection from the catheter being left in after surgery

All that said, the staff at the time did everything in their power to help me have the natural delivery but our daughter went into distress and my temperature shot up so we had to give up eventually.
Am due my 2nd in October and will be far more mentally prepared for the possibility that I will end up with a c-section, either planned for medical reasons or due to failed progression of labour.

I've had two emergency caesareans, the first wasn't too bad but the second one was prolapsed cord so it was really frightening. I wanted to have a caesarean for my second but the Doctor said my pregnancy was good and I was healthy but my gut feeling said 'push for a section', but the answer was "NO, go naturally". The Doctor should have listened to me but I wasn't a Private Patient!!!! Only for the brilliant Midwife on duty that morning our little man could have died or could have suffered brain damage, she is our son's saviour and we tell her that when we go and see her at work every April with our son. I find it hard to talk about this without getting upset. 6 months after this happened I sent my husband off for the snip, I just couldn't handle another emergency section!!! I bet the Doctor wished he had listened to me as he was there in the theatre and got a fair fright when the seriousness of this situation occurred.

- No one told me how much love I could have for another human being and that love would overcome any problems I had with my caesarean section. I had an elective CS and I had a full anaesthetic due to back problems (spinal wouldn't have worked). I cried so much knowing I wouldn't be awake or have my husband present when our long awaited (11 yrs) baby came into the world. I felt so hard done by and angry but in the end nothing matters just that the baby and

Mummy are healthy. The one problem we both can't forget is that my husband was outside waiting and was told he had a daughter but no one came out with the baby and when he spotted a nurse heading out with her coat he mentioned that he was waiting for the baby and she looked sheepish and said "oh wait here" and out she came with a bundle under arm and walked off. They obviously forgot to bring the baby out to my husband and so she didn't have Mummy or daddy cuddling her for the first hour of her life—way to go Rotunda!! Mind you I'd still go back there as overall their care was great....

- My section went very well but at the end when they're stitching me up, one of the Doctors or nurses (there were so many in the room!) said he was going to give me a suppository for pain relief. I said "sure no problem" and he wrote it up on my chart and went to get it but never came back!! My epidural wore off at the same time as my family arrived to visit the new arrival. I thought I was going to go out of my mind with the pain. The nurse looked at my chart and said she couldn't really give me anything because I'd had the suppository so recently. It was written up so as far as they were concerned it was given to me. I kept passing out and eventually a Doctor came and straight away gave me a morphine injection. It was a horrendous day.

  Also, on my first CS (the above was my 2nd), I reacted a bit mentally to the morphine and told the nurse that the baby was still inside me and the one in the cot wasn't my baby at all. I could feel my baby kicking inside me!! The nurse just tried to convince me otherwise and left. I thought that was a bit weird as I was obviously a bit mad and she left me in a room on my own with a newborn baby that I didn't want!!

- I had a baby almost two years ago by emergency c-section when his head wouldn't come down and they couldn't do anything to move my wee man.

I honestly believe they do not prepare women enough for this in ante-natal classes. I only had about 20-30 minutes talk relating to this in my classes.

I really could not believe how disabled I felt after the c-section. I got about 5 hours sleep before they woke me to 'get me moving'. I could not stand in the shower. Thank god there was a chair there. I also had my son with me the first night, not that I didn't want him I was just so so sore and zapped having been awake for around 43hrs.......!!

I also did not like the way breastfeeding was shoved in my face—I mean literally SHOVED IN MY FACE. I couldn't do it, baby didn't want it and I was too sore to sit comfortably and so when I went to the Midwife looking for a little bottle of milk to give me son she pushed me back to bed and said NO!! You're breastfeeding. When I said I wanted formula she refused me. Leaving me sitting with a crying baby until the Midwife came around in the morning with suppositories and asked why I was crying. I told her and she could not believe it and told me that I can feed him with formula and try breastfeeding again. It was like I had the plague with some of them when I said I was not breastfeeding. I know the advantages of b/feeding but my son has grown up to quite healthy and is bounding around regardless..... It should be taken into account about how sore women are after c-sections and I don't think some of them realise how sore it is.....I wish I'd known how swollen my legs would get and that they'd given me more than one pair of pressure stockings.....!! They were stinking..... But I cannot fault my Midwife who tried to help me deliver. She came to theatre with me and the theatre staff were brilliant. The anaesthetist was fantastic too. They did a really neat job of sewing me up too.....!! You should be told about the dreaded 'overhang' too.....

- Nobody told me anything much really!!! All the antenatal stuff was focussed on the normal delivery everyone expected to have.

At the end of the day, I've never been in labour and I had three non traumatic elective c-sections. All positive experiences, very much so. I didn't choose this; it chose me. My obs attempted several times to get my labour started but it didn't work, I was still just 38 weeks, the placenta had calcified, I was on blood pressure medication, I had a big baby and a small pelvis. Nobody told me how spaced out the morphine pump would make me. I refused to have it a second time and they gave me morphine via the spinal. I was sick the first time I had it, but not the second.

- Nobody told me that it would all be a little weird! In a good way, that's its very funny to see your husband in scrubs! The best piece of advice is wear cosy socks—yes you look like a nutter, but operating rooms are cold, and that most of all when you have your gorgeous little baby in your arms it doesn't matter how he or she got here, its still amazing and magical, enjoy every second.

- I had a planned section with my second baby. The date was booked months in advance, childcare for first child planned and all relatives ready. I went into hospital the night before on a rare hot summers night. I was told not to eat and drink that evening and was so hot I had to have a saline drip to prevent dehydration. I couldn't sleep with the drip, heat and excitement. Next morning I was all set to have a baby, only to be told to GO HOME as there were too many emergency/high priority sections that day. I had to do the whole thing again the next evening. Luckily I got my section the second day and my lovely boy was happy and healthy. Apart from this hiccup, my experience of sections as a public patient was positive. I had a planned section for medical reasons with first baby then chose a section the second time around. Have never gone into labour, but don't regret it for a second.

- Nobody told me that I would be in agony after my section because a nice chunk of the placenta had been left behind by the surgeon. I was in bits until I passed it the next day. The Midwife "forgot" to come back with my painkillers anytime I asked for some pain relief. Around 36 hours after my section I rang my husband to get him to bring me in the strongest painkillers he could get in the local pharmacy. I swallowed 8 of them the second I had them in my hand. I'll never forget the relief as the pain started to leave my body finally.

- I had a caesarean in Aug 2007. I was 15 days overdue!! I was induced on a Sat morning had another dose of gel six hrs later pains were unbelievable... my body went into shock from the labour well that's what they told me.. I was getting sick all the time, on the toilet... I couldn't sit or stand, ask for an epidural but they wouldn't give me anything because I hadn't dilated to 1cm. I was having pains but not progressing. Anyway on Sunday morning I had a show then they broke my waters!! I was just left to do my own thing.. they had me on the heart tracer I took it off and went outside for a cigarette—I couldn't even walk at this stage and there was a puddle after me from my waters. Some lady rang the phone in smoking room said come back in now... I was brought straight down for a section. I had the spinal block which was amazing!!! The baby had gone to the toilet inside and his heart rate was dropping and he was in distress... poor thing. They opened me at 16.16 and my little man was out at 16.19 he was so beautiful. He was 8lb 10oz. I didn't really get to see him he was brought to an incubator for 4 hrs I was left on my own in a room to recover for an hour or 2. He was jaundiced so they took him for me that night and that was great...

- I had an emergency caesarean and hospital staff in St. Lukes Kilkenny were brilliant. A friend of mine just had an emergency caesarean there on Friday and again thought staff brilliant BUT...and I find this shocking—the staff have now been told they are not allowed take baby from mother for a few hours on the first night, even if it is an emergency section because of new rules—this is terrible. The Midwives also feel terrible about this. Immediately after an emergency section you need this help as you just can't move!!!

- Nobody told me that you really don't care afterwards once everything is alright, your bub is safe and you are (in bits) but will be fine with time.

  Nobody told me what a fantastic, mostly underappreciated job our maternity services staff do, and how many people you can fit in an operating theatre, all just for little ole you and your imminent babs. I still can't pass the hospital without recalling the whole experience.

- Nobody told me that once the baby is born they show it to you and then both baby and your husband disappear without notice and you don't get to hold your little bundle.

  Nobody told me how friendly and reassuring the theatre staff would be. I had an emergency section as baby was huge, breech and I had gone into labour before my scheduled section date. Despite the emergency the staff all introduced themselves and helped make it a little less scary.

  Nobody told me that the company on a public ward would be great and the Midwives would be so helpful and feed my baby the first night.

  Nobody told me that the painkillers can cause diarrhoea, this doesn't mix well with an inability to move at any sort of speed.

- I didn't realise how disappointed I'd feel about not being able to deliver naturally. Especially after all the time, energy and indeed money I'd invested in being prepared for a natural birth: daily hypnobirthing practice, birth ball sessions, (the dreaded) perineal massage etc. But thankfully having all this knowledge gave me the confidence to persuade the Midwife to allow me skin to skin in theatre, which was absolutely brilliant, and made up for the total emotional trauma of the section.
  I didn't know I'd have to take my glasses off during the surgery. Cue panic!

- Hi, had an emergency C-section in 2007. I had complications at the end of a very easy pregnancy and I honestly thought I had lost my little one. I was so thrilled to hear her cry that day, I will never forget the euphoria. I was so thrilled that I never really noticed the pain, discomfort etc. I took any pain relief I was given in the hospital but found I didn't need very much by the time I got home. I found the whole thing very positive and would have no problem having another section if I go again.

- Nobody told me that you could get sever headaches from spinal block, this is caused by a pocket of air in your spine that doesn't fill back up, I had to go back to theatre to get what's called a blood patch done, this is where you get like another spinal and they take blood from your arm and put it in your spine

- I had elective caesarean as a result of diabetes....the worst part had to be the 4 failed spinal block attempts (I have strong tendons which kept bending the needle) so finally I got the epidural on try 5. But it was worse only because I started to tense up—if I hadn't I'd have been fine. I also had 4 cannula sites, one of which became swollen. I vomited on table but was told that is actually quite normal. Then I lost a lot of blood and went into shock—the shaking was strange. I did drive the nurses in recovery mad because I wouldn't sleep and wanted to hold my little boy so they let me go to ward after half hour. Then I suffered a serious infection (won't go into details) and was on IV antibiotic for 2 weeks. And after all that, I would do it all again tomorrow.....advice I would offer is: Don't be too proud—take the suppositories offered—they work wonders. Don't do too much when you are up and moving again. Bed to chair, chair to toilet should be enough for couple days. If you have staples expect the staple removal to be like a sting and hopefully you won't get too much of a shock. And, most of all, remember you have a wonderful baby as a result of it. Then go home and make your other half do everything for couple of days....well, it's worth a try.

- I had a emergency section 6 yrs ago found it very traumatic and still haunts me to this day

- Nobody told me that your breast milk can be delayed a further 24 hrs after a section.........it was defo true for me,....Also my section was an emergency and I hadn't got granny knickers packed..all other underwear rubbed on scar in hosp....

- I had 1 emergency section after a failed forceps delivery, heading for elective caesarean in Oct. I thought I'd never recover and feel normal again.....3-4 weeks makes such a difference!! For breastfeeding it can take a bit longer for milk to come especially after a traumatic labour resulting in a caesarean. This lead to a very irritable baby that I could barely deal with because was in too much pain to get baby out of the crib....a little bit of formula for the first night or 2 to top up baby will not be the worst thing you'll do and allows you feel a little sane. Some of the Midwives can be a bit militant about the breastfeeding and I can remember waiting for the night shift staff to come on so baby would get a top up. As far as I can tell it did no harm!! You bleed a lot, maybe I was clueless but wasn't expecting this to happen. I was getting through several nightgowns and PJ's a day, once they got stained I think you should be warned to take in black gear!!! Maybe that's vanity but for the next one that will be the plan!!

- I wish someone had told me how painful it is getting your staples removed. It was dreadful and wish I had been warned...... Also I have had 3 caesareans, 2 emergencies and one elective. All three births were completely different. Even if you have had one section the next may not be the same.

- Nobody really talks about c-section at all really do they? Everyone talks about vaginal births all the time and about epidurals and pain relief etc etc but you never hear people talking about c sections. I had an emergency caesarean (was induced on first child) and hadn't a clue what to expect. The thing that shocked me the most was the pain of recovery and the nasty overhang.

- I had an emergency caesarean section and found it very scary and traumatic being rushed down to the operating theatre. Luckily I had gone to antenatal classes and knew that there could be up to ten people in the room at any one time so this did not scare me when I got down there and the place looked packed. At all times the Midwives were great. I was terrified that when the baby stopped breathing he or she may have been hurt plus it was terrible that I was going to be awake for the whole thing. Thankfully it all went well. I am very active and fit and swam up until the morning of the birth but nothing had me prepared for the fact that I found it so hard to move after the operation. I didn't manage to get a shower until I got home as everyone seemed to busy to help me walk to the showers. Even a small walk was hard. Plus ... and this is the main thing I kept pressing the button for more morphine, thinking it killed the pain but...I got very sick on it and dizzy. I ended up getting sick twice and felt totally out of it! I wish some one had warned me of this and I wouldn't have been trigger happy on the button. I put myself under a lot of pressure to get moving quickly as everyone else seemed to be coping so well...

- Nobody told me that the epidural might fail during a section and I ended up feeling the whole operation.... horrendous stuff............

- After I had my 2nd section, on the 2nd day I got this awful pain in my shoulder, it was so bad and at times it felt like I couldn't breathe, I took painkillers but they didn't help and I thought there was something serious wrong but when I mentioned it to the nurse they told me it was a deferred pain from trapped wind which travels to the shoulder it's called something but I can't remember, so bring peppermint tea and water, it works a treat...
  Also recovery really isn't bad, the quicker you get out of the bed and moving slowly the better. For my 1st section I was unconscious for a few days and this felt like my first, I was so surprised at things.

- Nobody told me how nice it would feel to have shower once you are able to get up and about after an emergency section!

- Nobody told me that the epidural/spinal block (I've had both) would be so painful to get put in. It was the most agonising thing ever.... even with local anaesthetic.

- I was not told how much my legs would swell after the section. I had emergency section and I was unable to bend my legs for days because of swelling. My feet wouldn't fit into any shoes—for me was the worst part of having a section.

- Nobody said anything about the how much pain you can have afterwards with trapped wind. With my first section (emergency) I didn't do anything proactive to get bowels moving as didn't think it would be such an issue. And I was crippled with the pain of trapped wind for weeks afterwards worse than any other part of the recovery. I'm now just 11 days after my second section (emergency too) but I was very conscious of drinking loads of water, eating fruit and taking prune juice too. My bowels are still not back to normal but I think I've avoided that pain this time around. The food provided in hospital is totally unsuited to good digestive health—white bread, stodgy food and no fruit.

- I'm due my 3rd caesarean soon and nobody told me that after the 1st I would feel like I was stitched up too tight I thought I would never stand straight again plus I wasn't told you had to wear granny knickers after as I couldn't bear anything close to scar. I wasn't told I would feel like fainting during the operation plus thinking I was going to throw up. It cant be that bad as I'm doing it again.

- Nobody told me that epidurals can slow down labour. I thought they just took away the pain. Nobody told me epidurals don't actually last that long, but can easily be topped up. Nobody told me (well they did after section) that the staples are removed before you leave the hospital....a bare 4 days after you get them

- It's great to sit down and share my thoughts on my caesarean section that I had 5 ½ months ago. I'll start by giving the practical details of Stephen's birth. The hospital I was attending was Kerry General Hospital. I had been having bit of trouble with blood pressure being on the high side and very swollen legs during the last trimester. Our baby had been lying obliquely and my sister who is a qualified acupuncturist, had advised me to use Moxa sticks to help turn baby, which worked. However at 7 days over I had an appointment at the Clinic and I was told the baby hadn't engaged and was high and mobile, which in itself would not have caused a problem but my blood pressure continued to be a little high.

The decision was made to admit me and to see if my blood pressure would drop over the night but it stayed the same. I was told that I could not be induced because the baby was so high. The Dr could not have been nicer and explained my options and said he felt that there was a reason baby had not engaged.

The decision was made to section me at 10 days over although I had been practising hypnobirthing and really wanted a natural birth, I also felt that there are things in life you can't plan for and that a section was in the best interest for my baby. All the practical aspects of the surgery were explained to me in detail and I made it very clear that I wanted to breastfeed and knew that my milk would be slower coming in something I thought I was prepared for. When Stephen was born apparently the cord was wrapped around his neck twice meaning he never would have been able to engage and I was told if I had gone into labour in the cord would have tightened around his neck with each contraction causing him severe distress. For this reason I am eternally grateful that the decision was made to section me. As I said the practical aspects of the surgery were fully explained. What was never once mentioned was the emotional impact that having a section can have. When he was born I did shed a tear, and he was placed beside me however I was unable to hold him. He as then taken away to be weighed etc and my husband accompanied him to the nursery. They knew I wanted to breastfeed but I had agreed that if he was starving he could be given a small bit of formula as I told I would be in recovery for two hours.

This is the part I have huge issue with. I though it was normal for all hospitals but it appears many Mums are given their babies much earlier than two hours especially when breastfeeding. I had no complications in surgery so as far as I know this was just the hospitals policy. I remember being in recovery repeatedly asking to see my baby being told no I had to wait. They weren't even able to tell me his weight!! When I was finally allowed down to the ward, he was brought in and although I felt he was so adorable, if truth be told I felt like he could be anyone's baby, I didn't feel a connection.

It made me even more determined to breastfeed to help bonding and the nurses were great in helping him get latched on. I found breastfeeding very difficult and had to keep asking for help during the five days we were in hospital and although the Midwives were so obliging I felt like I was floundering. One day I fed him for pretty much seven hours straight and eventually the Midwives asked me would I like them to give him a small bit of formula while I slept which I did. Then I felt like the worst mother in the world for giving my baby formula! Although there is a lactation consultant in the hospital I was never asked would I like to see her (it didn't dawn on me to ask to see her unfortunately). At no time either was I encouraged to use a breast pump even though I had done my research before I went into hospital, all my info vanished when I had Stephen!

I eventually abandoned breastfeeding at two weeks which I really regret. I was also told I had to be flat on my back for 24 hours after the surgery and was unable to lift Stephen of change him etc. I had to ring for a Midwife if I thought he was hungry so they would lift him out of his crib and into my arms. I found it so hard to wind Stephen when I was unable to sit up and I think this was contributing to his feeding difficulties. After the surgery I was not given the morphine drip (I am not sure why, as I was told I would have it) but suppositories and tablets instead. I was in a huge amount of pain and when I was finally allowed to sit up and get up out of bed, I was doubled over and shuffling like a 90 year old.

Again I probably should have spoken up but I just assumed I had a low pain threshold which quite simply may be the case! I remember one time the nurse had swaddled Stephen and I could see the blanket was near his mouth and it took me very ounce of my strength to use the bed rail to pull myself over so I could pull it down. It was the sense on helplessness that was horrible in the 24 hours after the section it was something I was completely unprepared for. It has been so therapeutic to put my experiences down on paper and I would like to thank you for taking the time to read this. My intent is not to scare anyone but I feel if I having a section next time I would be so much better prepared. I really think the emotional consequences should be discussed in the hospital. I really thought I was the only one who had trouble bonding with my baby (something I never told anyone). It was not till I was talking to Mums on an online forum that I realised I was not alone. I think I also would be more assertive in getting breastfeeding help in the hospital.

▌ Emma Shanahan & Baby Stephen born April 2nd 2009

• I had an emergency c-section in May after a long labour. I was brought into hospital to be induced when I was 10 days overdue, I got two lots of gel and the next day I was 10 cm dilated and ready to push. My baby got distressed because his head couldn't come down far enough for me to start pushing and my temperature flew up so I was brought down to theatre.

What I wish I had known beforehand was: That they strap both your arms down to the table while in theatre, you are kinda like Jesus on the cross (only way I can describe it) one arm was hooked up to the monitor and the other to the epidural. I started to have a panic attack when they strapped me down as I wasn't aware they did this. Also they put a mask over your mouth and nose (might have been an oxygen one) because my arms were strapped down I couldn't remove it so started screaming with panic, they then took it off me. When they put the screen up I wasn't prepared for how close to your face it is, like I could literally see nothing at all in front of me.

I wasn't aware that the minute the baby is taken out and is checked over partner is whisked away with the baby and you are left all alone. This to me was the hardest part of all, I got a quick glimpse of our son and that was it for three hours later when I was brought back to my room. I was left on my own while I was being stapled and tidied up and this took about 50 minutes.

My obstetrician was talking to another Doctor, she seemed to be teaching him or something and I could hear phrases like 'not there, too near the bowel' things like that and it was sickening. Because I had an epidural I could feel everything although it wasn't painful, still you can feel the Doctor rummaging around inside you getting the baby out, I could feel her pushing back my ribs and I could feel this emptiness kinda like a hollow feeling once our baby was lifted out.

I think had my hubby still been with me I wouldn't have focused so much on what the Doctor was doing and wouldn't have felt so alone and scared. No one told me that you can start to shake violently once the baby comes out, I was so bad my shoulders were lifting off the table and my arms were hopping like mad, I was physically sick a few times as well and I have heard that this is fairly normal.

I wasn't prepared for how awful I felt once I came back to my room and my husband arrived back from the nursery with our baby. I couldn't move in the bed so couldn't hold him, I had to watch my husband struggle to change our baby's nappy on the end of our bed and I was desperate to get up and help him but couldn't. It was hard watching him feed our baby as well. I always imagined I would be the first to do these things. We had visitors that night and the next morning and I was still lying flat on the bed not able to move with the pain and stiffness so I felt so jealous of others getting to hold my baby before me. The night I had the section I couldn't get out of bed to feed our baby so had to ring a buzzer for the Midwives and I had to watch them feed, change, wind and settle my baby. All this is so hard to deal with I remember crying when I finally got to hold him and I used to whisper all the time to him 'I'm your MAMMY' I was so fearful that he was wondering where I was for the first 24 hours of his life. My bowel was in bits for days after the op, having lots of trapped wind, I remember my bladder was weird as well i.e. I got the urge to go to the loo very suddenly but once there nothing really came out, my Doctor explained all this was normal after surgery.

The big knickers is a huge thing, all the ones I brought to hosp were too painful as the band of them were sitting right on my scar, after a c-section you need panties that go right up to your belly button, I ended up sending my husband into Dunnes and he bought lots of size L boxer shorts for me and these did the trick wonderfully for about two weeks after!!!

For anyone who goes through a long labour and especially any-one that has been given the gel and has had a lot of internal examinations as well before having a c-section, be prepared for being very sore 'down below' for weeks afterwards as well as having to recover from surgery, its tough.

I bought the Gentlebirth hospital birth preparation CD at 20 weeks and I found it brill. I listened to it every day and found it so relaxing, I copied it to my ipod and found it great in hospital for the labour. However when I was brought down to theatre I didn't bring it with me, if I had I could have listened to it while I was on my own after my husband was taken away with our baby, it would have kept me calm and it would have taken my focus away from what the Doctors were doing. I don't know if I would have been allowed have it in theatre but if need a section on my next baby I will certainly be asking!!!!

I hope anyone reading this ends up being prepared for what's ahead. Looking back the only negative bits were just because I wasn't prepared/made aware of how it all works...how cold and strangely quiet the theatre is.......how you don't get to hold your baby for up to an hour afterwards while you're being stitched.. how painful it is the first time you get up out of bed after op (I had spinal block). I nearly fainted. How important it is for every Mum to be to read up on sections as I hadn't even contemplated it, thought I was young healthy and heading for a natural birth. You only get minutes in the case of an emergency section to try and take it in that your baby is in distress and you're having a section NOW! How important your partner's role is during and straight after a section. You won't be there for your little baby which I found heartbreaking. My daughter has such a strong bond with my husband and I'm convinced its because they got that chance to bond.

I didn't care whether I had a section or natural birth as long as baby and I were fine. I had two caesarean sections. I found it difficult in that you are still expected to look after your baby the day after you have the section—it is uncomfortable getting around. After the 1st section I was very tired for the first 6 weeks and couldn't consider driving. However, I think that that was because I had the baby with me.

On my second pregnancy opted for a section because our daughter had been diagnosed antenatally with a heart problem. I wanted to make sure that the teams and beds were prepped for her arrival. I was up and out of the bed and visiting my daughter in Crumlin hospital 24hrs after the section. I was a bit uncomfortable and tired but it was really no problem. I didn't have my baby at home at all and so recovered very quickly—actually within 2 weeks, forgot I'd had a section at all!

• I attended the National Maternity Hospital Dublin, Before having the twins I Found the hospital Excellent. I had a c section. The operation part was ok only felt pulling sensation. What I didn't like was when the first twin was delivered they didn't bring the baby over to me but the other twin they showed me for a second. After the operation I was in recovery room for over 24 hours and I was not allowed to see my babies which I found VERY upsetting. The Midwives wouldn't tell me anything either. After I was united with my babies I got very little help. I basically was left minding two babies. My husband ended up for 5 days coming into hospital to mind the babies so I could get some rest during the day. I wasn't offered any help to take the twins at night. My blood pressure was that high the Doctor demanded that the Midwives took them at night so I could get some sleep even at that I had to beg. It took me 6 to 7 weeks to recover. It was very painful but worth it!!

• I had an emergency cesarean section in April of this year. What nobody tells you is the whole panic of an emergency caesarean section. All the books and magazines prepare you for a planned one. It was the scariest 10 minutes of my life but worth it all as I now have a beautiful daughter. Nobody tells you about all the machines and drips you are hooked up to in theatre. That my hubby was not allowed in theatre....... the amount of people in theatre with you........ how doped you will be afterwards from all the drugs in your system.... how the Midwives station was down the corridor and I had to walk down there when ever I thought the pains were getting worse. (I had gone in the day before my daughter was born). Nobody tells you how important it is to have hubby/partner with you or that I wouldn't get to hold my daughter for a few hours after she was born. My husband brought her off to feed her. I don't think I missed out on the bonding. I wasn't in any real pain but just uncomfortable. Nobody told me how uncomfortable it is getting in and out of bed for really only the first day or so or how you have a lovely overhang of skin!!!! I still feel uncomfortable if I wear jeans all day. You can't wait to get home and get into track suit or PJ's. I didn't expect how helpful, friendly and professional everyone was. That you really don't know yourself until you hold your baby and that it was totally worth it all.
The reason why I had to have an emergency C- Section was that the placenta had moved away from the uterine wall and not enough oxygen was getting to the baby.

• I had an emergency caesarean section a few weeks ago. I'd planned to breastfeed, but after 2 days of trying, I found it too difficult (Firstly, I was in so much pain, couldn't have baby leaning against me or beside me. Secondly was so drained and weak from not being allowed to eat much for the first few days, needed the Midwives to give a cup feed at night).

I had to get the Midwife to lift the baby out of the crib to feed him with bottles. I found the hospital short staffed at night and so they were very impatient with me asking for help. My husband was allowed into theatre with me once it was all set up and he'd to wear a gown. They lifted the baby up about a tent-like screen to show us so we saw him immediately. I was surprised how painful the injection of spinal anaesthesia was and it felt like it took forever to get it into me. I got to do the skin to skin contact the next day.

It took up to 2 wks before I could stop taking pain relief. I felt I could have done with more pain relief the first few days in hospital but they were afraid they would overdose me! As I was pretty much restricted to the bed for the first few days, I'd a catheter inserted and I'd to get an injection each day to prevent blood clotting. Had to wear tight TED stockings (which I found itched me to death). One of the Midwives showed me how to bottle feed and burp baby...which seems daft but I really came from knowing nothing so I really appreciated that. I was worried about the pain of the staples being taken out a week later. It turned out it was absolutely nothing to worry about, I felt almost nothing. The public health nurse arrived out 2 days after we'd arrived home and we found her advice very helpful. I showed her where baby would be sleeping etc... and she had more up to date advice than what the hospital were doing.

I found the hospital generally good but think it would be better if they restricted visitors at night to spouse only as found it really noisy (and I was in a private room!)...plus, you've enough noise with trolleys of food, cleaners and Midwives walking about.

• There is lots of stuff that nobody warned me about c-sections. I've have 2 sections. The first was elective and second was an emergency section. For me I prefer the emergency as I felt I was a bit more a part of the birth.

Anyway one thing that someone did tell me was that after the baby was delivered and there was no problems with them don't let anyone else hold them except for Daddy. Don't let them clean them or dress them before you got to have skin to skin contact. For me that was when I felt like a mammy not when they lifted them out and held them up for me to see but when you get to have them place on your chest in all their glory !! The Midwives did try to dress them both times but I had my husband warned and he stood his ground.

Prior to the birth of my daughter I stayed away from all of these kinds of stories as I found there were more scary stories than anything else. I am sorry that some girls had horrendous experiences, however I'm also aware that some first timers will read these and be scared witless for no good reason. So, my experience and resulting advice is as follows:

I had an emergency c-section six weeks early as my waters broke and baby was in distress. The whole thing happened extremely quickly and I was not in the least bit prepared for it. I had been blithely doing yoga and aiming for a natural birth. I had a spinal block, which was not painful, and found the whole experience amazing from start to end and would have no problem doing it again. For the recovery I found the following helpful...

- After being in recovery drink plenty of fluids to ward off constipation and sleep as much as possible.
- Get up as soon as you can, even with catheter in tow. I had to go down to the NICU to see baby and managed it in a wheelchair around 9 hours after the operation. I think will power has a lot to do with it. The next morning I walked around. Walk around as much as possible.

- Take all pain relief on offer and request more if you have to. A Difene suppository for the first morning or two was enough to get me going. Continue to take pain relief at home for as long as you need.
- If you're breastfeeding sit in an upright chair and use a v-shaped cushion or two pillows and bend your knees and roll to get out of bed
- Don't be afraid to have a shower. The wound is numb so you won't feel anything. Also, you have to wet the dressing to remove it within a day of the operation. However, you will have to put the TED stockings back on afterwards, they were fairly disgusting.
Overall, I had a very positive experience. Can't say it wasn't pain-free but I never expected it to be no matter what route I took.

I had an elective caesarean in 2008. My baby was measuring very big and he hadn't dropped. The Doctor wasn't willing to let me go over and gave me the option of induction or c-section. I'm glad I took the section as babs was 11lbs.

▍ What did I wish I had known:

• That I would shake uncontrollably while lying on the table. It just freaked me out a little.

• That I would have to wear those awful surgical stockings afterwards—they are horrible and very hard to get onto extremely swollen ankles/legs.

• The amount of bleeding afterwards (I didn't realise it would be so much for so long)

• My baby was in Special Care and on the first day I expressed milk for him... it wasn't a lot and looked a strange colour (but its colostrum). A stupid Midwife threw it away because she thought it looked funny—I was devastated. The paediatrician told her when I brought the next lot down that it was fine that is the colour for the first few days. It was only then I discovered that she threw away the first lot!!!!

▌ On the Plus Side:

• I breastfed successfully within an hour of birth (lying down in the delivery room)

• Midwives were fantastic on the first night. I thought that I would be bothered by them having to change pads etc. They were great

• Take all the meds on offer and if they are not forthcoming keep asking for them. They helped with the pain.

• My baby ended up in special care after getting sick during the first night and he spent 48 hours in an incubator. A fantastic Midwife on night duty rang my mobile to get me to come down and breastfeed during the night. She was really supportive, really helped me and gave me the start I needed—It helped that it was quite and the middle of the night. I guess I got lucky!

• The stitches didn't hurt getting them out

• I had no problems getting the catheter out and moving after day 1 but I had the motivation that my baby was in Special Care—three floors away!

• I had a caesarean section 12 years ago. It was funny and terrifying all at the same time.
I had a problem with my liver (pregnancy related) so they knew my baby would come early, but they didn't know if it would be a natural birth or caesarean. Anyway my waters broke and I was taken into hospital and two weeks later I was brought down to have a caesarean. On that day I was brought to the

labour ward....hubby followed behind me with a few things... one of which was a spray bottle for when I was induced. When my hubby took out the bottle it was a spray bottle for spraying flowers....the Midwives roared laughing. They induced me within a half hour, that was at 9.30 am and at 7.30pm there was still no move on my baby and because I was losing so much blood, they wrapped me in what looked like tin foil...Jesus, I must have looked a sight.

An hour later the Doctor came in and insisted I needed a caesarean, I pleaded with her to leave it for just awhile, so she agreed to a half hour. Then they came back and brought me in to have the caesarean, I wanted my hubby with me, but they wouldn't let him come into the theatre with me, then they told me something that made me feel like I was in a horror movie. They were doing the caesarean while I was awake...I nearly went mad....in the end I had two nurses holding my hands while the Doctor cut into my tummy and I was wide awake, I was terrified....THOUGH I MUST ADMIT, I FELT NOTHING, AS I WAS NUMB FROM THE WAIST DOWN ! It was just the thought of it that frightened me so much. I was so frightened that I didn't get to hold my baby, the Doctor lifted him over the screen that stopped me seeing my tummy wide open and asked if I wanted to tell everyone what I had, but I was so frightened that I screamed that I don't care, I just wanted them to close me up. I have to say i got great care from Doctors and Midwives alike, but I was really unprepared for being awake during the caesarean and being wrapped up like a turkey!

• I had a c-section 3 months ago for the birth of my first child. Here is my story.

I was told at my 32 week scan that the placenta was low, and the Doctor may suggest a CS. The next scan was at 34 wks, and the placenta was still low, but nothing prepared me (nobody told me) that I would be booked into hospital at my 36 wk scan, which I attended alone. I was dispatched to the Doctor after my scan (it was always a different Doctor after each scan), 'bloods' were taken immediately, and I was told that they were finding me a bed that very night and I would not be returning home until after the birth. I was completely unprepared for this shock, had to ring my partner to come to the hospital with a bag packed. I spent the first night in the postnatal ward, the only pregnant woman in there, the others all new Mums. The shock of seeing some of the sectioned Mums brought in didn't calm my fears either. I ended up having to stay for 2 weeks before they decided on a date, which I didn't want. I had my heart set on a natural birth, but I was told I had placenta praevia, though they would never tell me what grade it was.

I was lucky that I lived within easy reach of the hospital, and after seeing my miserable face for a few days, my consultant agree to release me during day time hours, as long as I was collected and brought back each night. I can't say I was an easy 'patient', I didn't think my condition was serious, and kept asking questions, asking for scans on a weekly basis to see if there was any change in the placenta. To cut a long story short, was told I was having a caesarean at 38+3. I had never had a bleed, as was predicted with my condition. The thought of the caesarean terrified me, I thought I would die on the table, or something would go wrong with baby.

▌ Things I Wish I'd Known

• What Grade of Placenta Praevia I had, and my chances of a natural delivery.

• The incredible thirst I felt during op, was asking for my lips to be wet (they did oblige).

• How stiff and sore I would be afterwards.

• How long I would be bleeding afterwards.

• How to cope with new baby while recovering from surgery, i.e. breastfeeding, lifting, bonding, getting out of bed, all very major things when you are rendered almost immobile, and baby's needs must be met

Having said all this, the operation went well, and my daughter was delivered alive and well! My partner was allowed attend the op with me, which calmed me. Baby was held over screen for me to see, and then whisked away for injections, my partner ran after her, leaving me alone for the rest of the op. It took a strong mental effort to remain calm. I was told after the surgery that my blood loss was minimal, as I had been hearing of a possibility of a massive bleed this was a great relief. Overall, my stay in hospital was 3 weeks from start to finish

In hindsight, I did recover over the course of 2 months....although at the start I thought I never would. My baby is a joy to me now. Looking back, the experience doesn't seem as bad as it did then, but at the moment, I'm unsure whether I ever want to try again

Thanks for giving me an opportunity to tell my story. Therapy indeed!

• I also had a section in 2008 for placenta praevia. The Doctor told me at my 37wk check up that I would not be going home and was to have section at 39wks.

They brought me down to theatre at 8am as I was first on the list. My husband was brought in just before they started. My son's head had embedded in the placenta proving it very difficult for them to get him out. There was a lot of panic and the pressure I felt as they tried to get him out was huge. After what was basically brute force and use of forceps my son was born at 9.29am. (I had expected it to be all over at this stage.) My son was quickly taken by nurses as was slow to cry, he was very bruised from the forceps.. on his head, his side even his legs. They then handed him to my husband who held him beside my face for me to see. At this point I began to feel very weak and could feel the panic in the room. My husband was asked to leave and wait for me in recovery. The bleeding was excessive but thankfully with patience from my consultant he stemmed the bleeding though I had to have excessive stitching on uterine wall where vessels wouldn't contract.

My recovery was very slow, I was very bruised from the forceps, my blood count was 7 and I did not expect the pains after to be so severe. I've been told to expect to have placenta praevia again as the placenta may attach to the scarring low in the womb. But if I do have another section I'll be bringing my own stash of pain relief, instead of having to beg for a Panadol. Also I'll be more prepared for the pain from when they take out the drain... ouch!! They didn't give me staples but a 'bead' which thankfully was pain free to remove.

• I had a c section on my first born. I was just gone 20 yrs old. I was very scared as I had moved to Carlow to be with my boyfriend at the time. I was in a very bad relationship which put me in a lot of strain through the whole pregnancy. I am from Dublin and he was from Wales... He had his family living in Carlow also... Mine were all still up in Dublin.
I can remember waking up at around 8am with pains in my back. They were bearable but I was worried as I was not due for another 2 weeks time. When I told the boyfriend who was sleeping beside me. he didn't believe me so I was left to walk to the Doctors on my own, I never thought that I was in labour, so I just got up and waltzed down to the GP as if there was nothing really wrong.

When I got to the GP I remember sitting in the waiting room thinking of what I was going to make for dinner that evening. When I was called into the Doctor and he told me to lie down so he could listen to the baby's heartbeat I didn't really take any notice that I might of been in labour. But when he did say you're in labour you need to go to the hospital. I was like.. "are you serious??? I'm not due for another 2 weeks and the boyfriend wont believe me". The Doctor then rang my boyfriend and told him that I was in labour and funny enough he thought the whole thing was just a false alarm. As I walked back to our house on my own as the boyfriend was STILL in bed... (I'd be dying and he wouldn't have believed me) I rang my Father in Dublin, when I told him I was in labour he started crying. I was like "I'm ok don't worry"!! I then continued to ring my sister, mother and friends as I walked home.

It wasn't until I got back to the house and put my bag at the door (that I only packed the night before) that the boyfriend actually believed me... I can't really remember having bad pains. I was actually pretty cool about the whole thing. When we arrived at the hospital and they checked the baby and that everything was fine.... I was in slow labour. I was gutted as I was starting to feel rather ill. I told him to go home as he wasn't much use anyways!! During that evening I decided to go for a walk around the hospital. I've never been in hospital before so I kinda hadn't a clue where I was going... But on my travels I ended up at the delivery suites. Dread came into my mind as I could hear the roars of some poor woman giving birth and it made me feel queasy. With that I ran into a spare room and started to vomit everywhere. Just my luck as I was cleaning up my mess a Midwife walked by the room and then came back into me to see if I was ok. By then I was starting to get painful contractions. She brought me into one of the delivery suites and asked me if I wanted to try some gas and air. I was like yeah ok sure why not. I took a little bit and the Midwife said I wasn't taking enough. With that I took a huge deep breath of the gas and air and I vomited everywhere. Thankfully the Midwife found the funny side of it though.

I must have drifted off on the bed in the delivery suite. I woke up at around 6 am. I forgot where I was for a moment and looked and seen a hospital gown on and rolled my eyes and said to myself "still here... jeez!!"

Then I felt this gush of water and looked down and was like eww!! I rang the bell for the Midwife to come and she asked me was I ok... I said to her " Either I have wet the bed or my waters have broken" with that she let out a giggle, and said they have broken and she brought me into the main delivery suite... By now I was getting really scared as I was in Kilkenny—a far cry from Dublin to where my family was and a fair distance away from Carlow to where my boyfriend was.

At around 10 am after I was changed into the gown I wanted to wear for labour and after they rang my parents and tried numerous times to ring my boyfriend whom they eventually got through to at around 11am... he was in work the dork... They all arrived then around an hour and a half later—just after I'd gotten the epidural for the labour. I was getting all geared up and ready when the Midwife was checking to see how much I was dilated she had a frown on her face. I looked at her to ask what's wrong and then she and another Midwife then called down around 4 consultants and Doctors to examine me. I felt so horrible and scared I wished and cried for it all to be over. They then told me that the cord was wrapped around the babies shoulder and it's starting to cut off oxygen and I needed to have a caesarean section. I started to panic. Thankfully my Father was in with me at the time and he helped me prepare for it, I begged them to give me a general anesthetic as I would totally freak out if I was awake when they cut me open and thankfully they agreed.

All I can remember from that is been wheeled out of the room and down to the theatre and my Father had tears in his eyes. When I woke up I was on the skinniest bed I've ever been on in my life I was told I had a 7lbs 15oz baby boy. I was soooo shocked—they told me that I was having a girl!! Whooops!!! But all the same when I saw him I knew that he was mine.

I have a huge scar going from one side of my stomach to another, I had a speedy recovery from the caesarean section. I hate the fact that I had to stay in the hospital for 5 days afterwards. But policy is policy. I had a natural birth second time round.

• I had an elective section on my 1st in 2006 and for me it was absolutely the right decision. I had made up my mind early enough into pregnancy that it was the road I wanted to go down and my Consultant was fully behind my decision. So the whole pregnancy was great as I knew exactly what was ahead of me. I was scheduled to be brought to theatre a week before my due date but turned out that my water broke 4 days earlier than planned, a Saturday afternoon. My husband was in Dunnes getting dinner for that evening and I called him to get me to hospital. We drove there with the bags not really knowing if I was going to have a section so I was a bit nervous. (I never did any classes so I knew nothing about giving birth) The Midwives at the hospital were lovely, they told me waters had definitely gone and baby had to come out. As I never actually went into labour I was offered to be induced or to have an emergency section. I chose the section. The whole experience for me was great. In the theatre everyone was so lovely. The scariest part was the spinal block because I didn't know how it would feel, but a lovely Doctor told me to lean on him and I wouldn't move. It felt like a bee sting and then my whole lower body started to feel numb straight away, even before I had lain down. It was funny because I remember trying to lift my legs to swing them around onto the bed and in my mind I was swinging them up but they weren't moving.

The Midwife had to move them. Weird!! Then, obviously I had to be shaved down there, but couldn't see anything or feel it so made no difference, and also had to have the catheter put in, but again didn't feel it so wasn't bothered. My husband was brought in then and he sat by my head. We chatted while the Doctor got ready, then she started and within no time at all I was told I had my beautiful daughter. She was placed on my cheek for skin to skin contact and I started to talk to her and she stopped crying. They held her there for what seemed like a long time before she was taken to be cleaned and I was stitched and cleaned up. My hubby was able to hold her and give her 1st bottle and I was wheeled down to my room. He came with me and we stayed there late into the night until the Midwives told him at 11pm he'd have to go so they could wash and dress me. Again, that was a bit weird having a bed bath and knickers put on, but to be honest I was so happy to be a Mum and have my baby girl I just didn't care. Nothing would have upset me that night. I didn't sleep a wink all night just stared at my baby and called friends. The next day I was asked if they could take out the catheter, which was quick and stinging for a while but I was asked to get up and walk to the bathroom and do a wee. I'm glad they did because I realised I was able to get up and move around and I didn't want to stay in the bed all day. So on Sunday evening when visitors arrived I was sitting in a chair and feeling great.

I stayed in hospital until Thursday, but had my own room and hubby was there most of the time anyway. By the following Saturday I was out walking and pushing the buggy.
I can't honestly say, for me it was all mind over matter. I knew what I wanted and was calm about the experience. I was determined not to let the operation leave me bed ridden so I got up early to move around. Getting the stitch removed pinched a bit but nothing too bad.

The only thing I really wish I had been told, or better understood about a section baby was that as she hadn't come down the birth canal all the mucus was not pushed out of her lungs. Although she was suctioned at the delivery, the following day a build up of mucus blocked her airway and she went blue. Luckily we were alert and watching her and were able to call the Doctor. She is 3 now and a healthy intelligent happy kid. I am expecting baby number 2 and am planning on another section. My only worry this time around is the hospital stay and being away from my daughter, and also I won't be able to pick her up. We'll see, I'll just have to be careful. I say good luck to anyone who opts for a section, it was a great experience for me and I wouldn't change a thing.

• I'm a first time Mum (my son is 5 weeks old) and I just thought I'd share my experience. My son was due on August 30th but no sign so on Sept 1st I went to my consultant's appointment and was told I'd be going in the following week to be induced. While I was pregnant, he was breech until week 37 and so all along I was told I'd be getting a planned caesarean if he didn't turn. Anyways he did so I thought ok no worries I'll just go with normal delivery. Boy was I wrong!! I went in to get induced on Tuesday Sept 8th and they gave me the gel at 4pm. By 9pm I was getting pains and at midnight they gave me a second dose of the gel. I was up all night then as the pains were getting progressively worse but my waters were still intact.

At 8am the next morning the consultant came to see me and said that I'd be getting my waters broken that day. In my naïveté I presumed I'd be heading to the induction room at (Cork) shortly but little did I know that I was at the mercy of there being an available bed in the induction room (by the way there's about 7 delivery beds to cater for all of Cork and its surrounding areas!). So there I am in agony all day and finally brought down around 5 to get the waters broken.

So they broke the waters and the contractions were coming thick and fast but no progression (I was still at 1cm since the night before). I have to say the Midwives were so lovely and so kind that they made the experience a bit better. By 10.30pm that night it was decided I'd go on the oxytocin (I think that's what it's called) drip and then the fun really started. My contractions were 4mins apart and incredibly strong.

They checked me again at midnight having increased the flow of the drip and brought me down for an epidural. The relief of the epidural lasted all of one hour. From then on I felt every contraction as well as a burning sensation from the catheter (this worried the Midwife when I said it). The night wore on and it was clear that the epidural was not working. By 6am I was in bits and the Midwife was trying to argue it with the registrar that I was in distress and something needed to be done. His response was to say that I could easily go another few hours on the drip and to prove his point proceeded to take blood from my unborn son's head to prove that he was not in distress at all. At this point the Midwife got mad and told him he could do his own tests as she was having no part of it as it was clear that I wasn't progressing and the more they upped the drip the more resistant my son was to it.

By 7am I was 3cm dilated and the opening to my cervix was thickening instead of thinning out. In fairness to the Midwife she waited until the shift change at 8am to ask another Doctor to sanction a section as she knew she was going to get nowhere with the registrar. By 8.16am my son was born. I was on enough painkillers at this point to floor an elephant so found picking him up and feeding him (breastfeeding) no problem. This all changed when I got home. Before I left the hospital I'd asked for a prescription for more pain relief. I was met with the response of "Really? Do you think you'll need it?" In my naïveté I thought ah sure maybe I'll be grand but how wrong I was. His first night at home, he woke around 2am for a feed. It took me 10 minutes to get upright in the bed and I was practically howling in pain. Then it took another few minutes to get him positioned on the breast and as he was a big baby the pressure of him on my abdomen was unreal.

I managed breastfeeding him for about 10 days before I had to stop from pain and exhaustion. Added to this emotionally I felt like a complete failure like I couldn't look after my own child. I'm actually welling up thinking about it. For the first 3 weeks I felt more like a childminder than his mother as I felt I had no bond with him. I'm getting better now but it was so hard in the beginning. I wish someone had told me that bonding takes longer after a section, that I would be in a world of hurt physically and that breastfeeding would be so hard. It kills me that I had to stop and maybe there's those out there that had a caesarean and breastfed just fine but unfortunately that was not my experience.

Our Positive Caesarean Birth

I was admitted to WRH at 38 weeks with 'unstable lie'—not a pure breech position with bum down, but feet dangling down. She remained breech that weekend, head down but very high on the Monday, transverse on the Tuesday morning and yet again breech on the Tuesday evening (I knew she had been the most active baby I had carried but I didn't really quite HOW active! I was at first very disappointed and scared at the thought of a section after two normal births but I must say, we managed to make the whole experience very special and memorable. I had practiced the Gentle birth CDs all along and I must say they really really did help, from the time the news of possible section hit me, through the night before, visualising it as a positive experience and it really did turn out that way.

We shared the evening before talking about our future with the baby we knew we would meeting the next morning and planning everything we wanted after the actual birth. The next day, after a lovely relaxed stroll into theatre, smiling and calmly greeting all the ante-natal Midwives, I became momentarily a little overwhelmed on entering the theatre because I had been zoned in a slow, calm place, which operating theatres are not.

It would have benefitted me to know a little more detail of everything about the procedure immediately on entering the theatre and so, for anyone else facing an unanticipated section for the first time here it is. I was asked many questions to check identity and whether I agreed and understood the need for a section etc, partner is not allowed to be present during preparation which I wish I had known beforehand so it wouldn't have taken me by surprise. They took off all but my nightie, added a blood pressure cuff, stuck on pads on your chest and back for heart monitoring, ask you to stand on a step to reach bed, added another step to bring knees higher and placed me in bent over position to receive anaesthetic. All of this happens in about 5 minutes, with about 10 staff in the theatre. I felt a tiny scratch for the one that numbs the site but nothing whatsoever for the administration of the actual spinal block needle, and within seconds I felt a lovely warm sensation down the back of the legs and into my feet, then they lifted my legs for me onto the bed and put up the screen to stop me seeing anything. (I know that if it wasn't for Gentlebirth, this would have been the point at which I felt my control being lost and panicked).

However, I used deep breathing, visualised my desert island stroll on the sand and focussed on staying calm. At this point, my partner appeared next to me with more reassurance, and I listened to every word between the staff about the imminent birth of my baby. It seemed like literally seconds before the lovely anaesthetist told me she was being born. All I felt was a lightening of the tummy as the fluid released and then she was lifted out (leg and arm first as she was lying across me). Seconds later I saw her and then as they explained, dad followed her into the recovery area for her checks and drying. Partner then brought her back in to show me as they were closing my wound. It took about 40 minutes to complete that, and hearing their conversation that all was well, added to the reassurance, so much so that I was chatting to the staff about all sorts, ecstatic about the birth, knowing that my precious bundle was next door enjoying skin to skin contact with dad snuggled into his chest as mine was not possible, just as I had requested, instead of a heat lamp.

A few more checks, then onto the post natal ward to reflect on the whole procedure which I can honestly say was the most calm, beautiful experience of my life. Yes, a different way of delivery, but certainly not the huge awful threat as some would portray it, and in my case, there was no question about opting for it rather than possibly endanger the life of my baby. For those Mums who find themselves in a section dilemma, I promise you that Gentlebirth preparation is a huge advantage, and the privilege of preparing for things to be the way you want them to a certain extent is also a bonus. It would never have occurred to me to request skin to skin with Dad, but thanks to Gentlebirth, that was a lovely aspect. The pain relief and relaxation techniques also helped greatly during the recovery. Our gorgeous daughter, Francesca Maria is also such a calm, relaxed, excellent feeder and contented baby. Good luck to all those Mums who are facing a section—draw your own special memories from doing it as much as you can the way you want to, and yes—enjoy it!

The consultant cautioned me that the recovery is much worse; everyone commiserated with me on hearing it was to be a section and warned of the recovery. Well, yes, the first two days are not the most pleasant, but neither were my previous 2 VBs and the Midwives were always on hand to help baby onto breast, lift from cot to me, and anything else you need. Partners can be present for 12 hours a day to help with washing etc if you wish, and by day 3 I found I was quite mobile and independent, stitches out and home on day 4 in no more pain than with a vaginal birth, just in a different area!!

The Midwives commented between themselves on the fact I didn't have pain relief on my last night in hospital and they hoped I would be OK and left me to sleep instead, and neither did I insist on a pain relief prescription to go home with. I am convinced that the power of the positive thinking and calm confidence from my CDs and GentleBirth reading really made for a faster recovery. She is 6 days old today and we are just back from a gentle 20 minute stroll in gorgeous sunshine with our little miracle, and as I will be 42 myself next week, I am soooo grateful to be enjoying my second chance at being a Mummy!

A big thank you to the staff at WRH for their wonderful care and support.

Jayne

- I think that c-sections get a bad rap generally by natural birth campaigners. I have been blessed with the birth of three children, all by section and all miracles. I have never dilated by more than 2 cm (even after 30 hrs of labour pains) and my first two children went into foetal distress several times, (in the absence of oxytocin). My first two labours ended in the race to the theatre, so I elected for the third one to be section from the start. All three births were beautiful, even in the midst of trauma; I am an example of someone who would have died giving birth 50 yrs ago. I have no doubts about that. Thank God for medical intervention. I don't need a calm yoga-esque experience I just needed my children to be born safe and well.

- I have two gorgeous children and both were born by section. My first was my daughter for "failure to progress". As far as I was concerned I was two weeks behind what the hospital scan stated, so when they brought me in to be induced at their 42 weeks, I was only 40 weeks per my dates. I was told I would have no chance of a vaginal birth as cervix was too high and hard. Booked in for the section to be told in the pre-labour ward that no, I had to go through full induction first. Went through the lot and got an epidural in the labour ward to cope. When the consultant decided that I wasn't getting anywhere he said we'd have to have a section. As this was my first and this is what we had turned up for I happily agreed. They gave me an epidural anaesthetic for the op. Everything was going fine, my daughter was born and while they were showing her to me (no skin to skin!) I started to feel that I had stopped breathing. I couldn't take a breath at all and started to panic. Some guy tried to calm me down and put an oxygen mask on me but that just made me feel like he was trying to suffocate me. He tried to point out the monitor that showed that I was breathing but I couldn't see straight I was in such a panic.
He told me that the epidural block had gone all the way up to the top of my neck and that was why I felt I wasn't breathing—you need to feel the muscles in your neck working—this was news to me. They couldn't raise me up as they were still stitch-

ing me and it was only when I got into recovery and I was elevated and the epidural starting to drain down that I felt better. My partner got an awful shock too as we both thought I was in severe trouble. No-one told me prior to getting the epidural that this could happen; at least if I'd been informed I may not have panicked.

My new son is just 4 weeks old today and he was an emergency section as he went into foetal distress and I started to bleed due to the placenta coming away. And I was so close to a VBAC! Ah well, he's safe and well as am I so I actually feel a lot better about this section than the first one!

• My cesarean section first time round was a nightmare. I went into hospital two weeks early after my waters broke, and they left me until the following morning as nothing was happening, after trying to induce me still baby wasn't ready to come. I was becoming scared and baby was in distress so they gave me an epidural but it wouldn't work, then gave me a second and that wouldn't work so they called in a specialist from another county to give me the third as at this stage I had to have a c-section, he informed me it had worked so I was brought down to the operating room, while they prepared me for the section, they sprayed this cold substance on my stomach to ensure that I couldn't feel anything below my stomach but I did and told them so but the same specialist said I couldn't so they began to cut and I screamed as I could feel the knife going through my body and nearly passed out with the pain, they told my husband to leave the room and gave me a general anaesthetic to put me out and when I woke up I had a baby boy, but I felt awful and couldn't bond with him at all for a few months as I was traumatised by the whole event. It took me three years to have another baby and I had to have another section but this time round they decided to give me a spinal block and it worked out much better. It just goes to show that when you are a first time mother giving birth, you are the mercy of the professionals in a hospital and take their word as gospel.... I feel very hurt and let down that this has happened to me and my son. I hope my experience will never re occur again.

• I knew I was having an elective c-section for 3 weeks before my due date. My obs didn't want to let me go over my due date due to ''special baby', PCOS and big baby.

I accepted it and felt calm about it, wanted my baby so bad and just wanted him born the safest way for him. I thought I was ok with it but after the birth I did feel sad for quite a while that I had to have the c-section. I think women who have not had a c-section see it as an 'easy' option—it's the whole 'too posh to push' mentality. Can I just say that I know some people have a long recovery from vaginal births, but having your abdomen cut open and your muscle wall is no walk in the park!

I found the birth experience quite relaxed and nice. I was calm about it and excited to see my baby. My spinal took a while to do but I found the staff in Wexford General fantastic and we were actually joking and stuff.

The anaesthetist did ask me to tell him if I felt sick and I did and then was sick, which I really wasn't expecting, but he gave another shot of something and that took that away right away. The anaesthetist spoke to me the whole way through and told me what was going on and distracted me when my baby and husband had left the theatre. I really appreciated that.

Things nobody told me? I'm going to change that around and say things people told me that I found really really helpful.

Whether you have a vaginal birth or a c-section, not every woman bonds with her baby immediately. My baby was in special care when I got back to the ward and I didn't see him properly until next day. It took me until day 3 to bond, but I knew I loved him but didn't have that overwhelming flood until a few days later. I knew this could be normal and was able to not feel guilty about it which really helped.

I only started breastfeed on day 2 and in the Special Care baby unit. The nurses there were fantastic and showed me a breast massage to do to help encourage the milk to flow. This is fantastic and I would recommend it to anyone. You massage the breast in small circular motions all around the nipple and then with the side of your hand you firmly push down from base of breast towards nipple as if pushing milk towards nipple. If you do this for a minute or 2 before trying to breast feed for the 1st few days until milk comes in it really helps. For breastfeeding I found that getting up and sitting upright in chair with feet slightly raised, using a breastfeeding pillow was most comfortable and pain free way to breast feed.

Make sure that you keep pain medication up. Do not let levels drop, so that if you feel ok and they offer you pain relief, take it! Take it every 4 hours because it is easier to keep pain at bay then it is to get rid of full on pain due to lack of pain relief. (It made me so mad for those poor women who felt they had to self medicate. I'm so sorry you were treated in such a fashion—I had to go to the Midwives station a few times because I was forgotten about during medication rounds).

Keep the wound as dry as possible. I did shower daily and washed the area but pat dry and best tip was to us Maternity Pad on the wound—it helps pad it and keep it dry! It was fantastic and stayed in place thanks to floppy belly and granny knickers! They are your friend after a c-section!

▍ Things no-one told me.

That I could stop using the surgical stocking/tight thingies once I was up and moving (which was next morning—up and down to special care!). Trying to get them on after a shower was horrible!

How much I wished my husband could be with me all the time to help out with baby.
To avoid hearing funny stories or jokes for the 1st few days!! Laughing was a confusing mix of wanting light relief and pain!

Not to get dressed in bathroom with door open to room while priest is doing Communion rounds!!!!!

How much better you feel when you make yourself get up and about and how proud you are that you can do it.

How glad you will be to get home!

How you need help at home for a while.

How it can be a really positive experience and a c-section doesn't always have to be a negative thing.

* Nobody told me that my life could be hell after my section. I just wanted to tell you about my side affects from having a c-section 2yrs ago.

I have severe nerve damage which I have lost count of how many medications and pain patches I've been on to help with the pain. I've even had steroid shots which only lasted 2 weeks. I'm in the pain clinic every 2 weeks still trying every medication in the book with no joy.

Here is what I can't do or have problems with.
When my bladder fills up I have pain
When my bowls move I can't move an inch with the pain
I can't have sex cause it's to sore
I can't push my child in his buggy up even a slight hill
The playground is a nightmare with all the lifting up and down
Wearing heels kill me

Certain jeans that put pressure on my scar I can't wear
General cleaning (hovering, making beds etc)
Any many many more. So I wake up in the morning with pain
and go to bed in pain. I'm always narky cause I'm always in
pain. The drugs make me sleepy and forget full and still only
scratch the surface with the pain. My stomach goes into spasms
even without doing anything to aggravate it. This leaves me
screaming crying with pain not being able to sit or stand with
it. And because it's my nerves going into spasm it affects other
nerves in my body so the pain isn't just in my scar area. This can
happen up to twice a week. Due to all this I now have depression and battle with that every day too. So that's it, I will be in
pain for many years to come if not forever.

• My section was an emergency and I can't regret a second of
it because my son was in trouble and he needed to get out. I'd
have pushed him out through my nose if I had to! But the after
care was awful.
I was a private patient and left to cope in a room on my own.
Was climbing in and out of bed with my sore stomach, lifting
him, trying to breast feed while trying to lift the back of the
bed up and arrange the pillows behind my back myself. Agony.
Staff shortages meant ringing the bell wasn't particularly encouraged. My husband stayed with me all day to help and used
to nearly be in tears leaving me at night because he knew what
lay in store for me. Breastfeeding never fully took off for us and
I blame both the section drugs and the after care. The drugs I
can't help but the after care was just awful.

• My story is that I had emergency CS on my baby's due date
to her being distressed and me not progressing. I have to say
I found it ok...the worst part was not meeting my baby until
10am the next day...she was born at midnight, as she was in
ICU. I had to get out of bed and go to ICU to see her and I never
looked back. My husband wheeled me down (catheter in tow!!)
and I walked down after that. What I wish I'd known:

1. that there are good experiences of CS...I'd heard nothing but dreadful ones until I met a lovely woman in the ward before I was induced who'd just had one and she told me all about it...knowledge is power!!

2. That you have an overhang over your scar

3. That you bleed the same as a vaginal birth for a few weeks after

4. That there will be about ten or twelve people in the theatre...surgeon, Midwives, paediatricians, etc (woman above told me that so it didn't freak me out when I saw them all)

5. That taking out the catheter wouldn't hurt the way I thought it would (again others had told me that).

▌ Daniel's Calm Arrival

I was two weeks overdue and going in to be induced on Friday morning. The consultant had tried to break my waters on the Tuesday but said I was totally unfavourable and that I could wait a little longer if I wanted but they seriously advised against going past two weeks which I was in agreement with. I was glad to finally be going but I was a little disappointed at having to be induced as I felt going in naturally was really important if I wanted to achieve my VBAC but I decided just to be positive, use my Gentlebirth affirmations and to take in every minute of our special day.

My hubby and I headed off to CUMH early in the morning and got settled in. I just chilled out listening to my affirmations and practicing my breathing. I was examined at 10am and they said I was still unfavourable to have my waters broken but also that because I was so overdue using gel was too risky so the only way forward now was a c section.

I was really disappointed that my VBAC was not going to happen particularly as I was so looking forward to a natural empowering experience and hoping for a quick recovery.

We were booked for a section that afternoon and had to wait in the induction room in the meantime.
My husband was totally great he consoled me and was really understanding and negotiated a few things with the consultants for me. He made sure they knew that we wanted to be together throughout the procedure and that I wanted to hold the baby first. I had so wanted to feel involved in the birth this time as with my daughter the emergency section was very cold and clinical.

For the afternoon I tried to relax and I used the affirmations 'I am ready for whatever path our birth takes' and 'the safe arrival of my baby is the most important thing to me'. The theatre was really calm, the staff really respected my wishes that I wanted things relaxed and quiet; they spoke gently and explained things to me slowly. We were able to watch the birth on a TV in the theatre so we got to see Daniel coming out of my belly. The cord was wrapped round his neck four times, around his chest once and around his legs. As we didn't know we were having a boy, the consultant held him up to the camera so I was able to discover he was a boy for myself rather than being told. Daniel was cleaned up and the Midwife helped me hold him to my chest—it was perfect. She then brought the placenta over for me to see it; the cord was over three feet long which I was told is more than twice as long as the average.

I felt really glad that we went for the section, it was the safest option particularly in hindsight seeing the cord around him the way it was. I am so grateful to the staff at CUMH they made me feel so involved despite the need for surgery. I was so glad that my husband spoke to the staff so that I could hold Daniel first and that they let me announce his sex and see the afterbirth.

Sorry I've gone on, just wanted to give as much detail as possible as I know how much reading these stories helped me leading up to the birth. I would also encourage all the other VBAC Mums that although I didn't achieve my VBAC and have been really disappointed by this at times, I found what was more important was that I felt calm. I'm thrilled with little Daniel who was born weighing 8lb 15oz am so glad to be back at home where we're all getting to know our new family member.

Chapter III

■ Caesarean Birth—Why All the Fuss?

If you've had a positive caesarean birth experience or are satisfied that your caesarean was necessary you probably wonder what all the fuss is about when it comes to news reports about the increase in caesarean births. Caesarean births have increased 80% in the last 10 years. There's no doubt that caesareans can save lives but this staggering increase has a serious negative impact on the health of both mother and baby. This increase has not improved outcomes. In the absence of a medical condition a spontaneous vaginal birth is always the safest option for Mum and baby—that's worth repeating—in the absence of a medical condition a spontaneous vaginal birth is the safest option for you and your baby. Thankfully it is very rare for a mother or baby to die during labour but this has more to do with to with Mums being healthier, having smaller families, getting free antenatal care, antibiotics and hand hygiene in hospital. We know this is true because in other countries with lower caesarean rates than ours it is not at the cost of lives...their outcomes are in fact better than ours.

It's no news to anyone that Ireland is still experiencing a growing baby boom—around 75,000+ babies were born in 2009 and those numbers are likely to increase. Recessions and baby booms tend to go together.

The number of births between the 3 Dublin hospitals are skyrocketing—each hospital is gearing up for approximately 10,000 births per year and there are only 30 delivery beds. 30 delivery beds—now do the maths, consider what that could mean for your experience of giving birth. In a recent Irish Times story the caesarean rate within the 3 Dublin hospitals continues to grow particularly if you are a private patient. In the Coombe hospital. 1 in 3 private patients will have a caesarean birth compared to public patients where it's about 1 in 4. Private patients attending NMH are more likely to have give birth by caesarean also. The Rotunda's numbers are more evenly matched between public/private/semi-private.

To put it mildly we're in a bit of a quandary. Like every other nation that's trying to reduce it's caesarean rate we can't just turn back the clock—we have to figure out ways to make normal birth a more positive and safer experience for Irish mothers. The good news is we don't need to reinvent the wheel or even build bigger hospitals. (We need cleaner hospitals that's without question). There's already a mountain of evidence in how to increase normal birth rates—we just need to start using the evidence. At a grassroots level we need to change how we care for women during pregnancy and birth and encourage more women to explore their options and get second opinions.

In theory the answer is quite simple—putting it into practice is another story altogether (and for once it's not something that needs huge financial investment). But as you'll see old habits die hard....

▎ Caesarean Rates—It's a Numbers Game.

I won't try to dazzle you with statistics but this is important background information to have. The World Health Organisation states that there is no justification for any region in the world to have a caesarean rate over 15%. Despite what some Obstetricians think the WHO recommendations are not just for Third World countries and the WHO recommendations are not out of date. As a country's caesarean rate goes above 15% more women die. Caesareans are associated with 45% of all maternal deaths in the US. Would you be surprised to learn that your maternity unit may have an emergency caesarean rate of over 60%?

In his book 'The Caesarean', Obstetrician Dr. Michel Odent writes:

"The primary objective should not be to reduce the rates of caesareans: it would be dangerous, if not preceded by a first step. This first step should be an attempt to promote a better understanding of birth physiology and particularly a better understanding of the basic needs of women in labor. In hospitals where the watchword is to reduce the rates of caesareans, the first effect is usually an increased number of difficult births by the vaginal route and of dangerous last-minute emergency caesareans. This is exactly what we should avoid in the age of the safe caesarean. I have had many recent reports of deliveries during which the obstetrical team tried "everything" in order to avoid a caesarean: drip of synthetic oxytocin, epidural anaesthesia, and, finally, either a forceps delivery with episiotomy or even a caesarean after trying the use of forceps. Forceps have their place in museums. The last time I used forceps was in February 1965"

▌ How Do I Know If My Caesarean Is Really Necessary?

You might be thinking—"of course my caesarean *was/is* necessary." We need to consider what the indications are for surgical birth—as you'll see there's quite a big grey area.

You might be surprised to learn that the absolute indications for a caesarean birth are not very common but depending on your caregiver his absolute indications for a caesarean birth may make this list significantly longer (but they are most likely NOT based on current international recommendations).

Absolute indications for a caesarean would be:
• Your baby is lying sideways: Most babies arrive head first—basic physics here...a sideways lying baby is most likely not coming out the traditional route. But this is assuming you've been offered a manual turning (ECV) and you may have more options available to you if this isn't your first pregnancy.

• True CPD: The accurate definition of cephalopelvic disproportion (CPD) is when a baby's head or body is too large to fit through the mother's pelvis. True CPD is very rare, but many cases of "failure to progress" labours are given this diagnosis. When an accurate diagnosis of CPD has been made, the safest type of birth for Mum and baby is a caesarean delivery. The problem is that true CPD can't be diagnosed until labour is already underway. Looking at your hips (or shoe size) or basing your baby's size on a digital photo can not diagnose CPD. It is very rare for a healthy non-diabetic woman to grow a baby that is too large to give birth to. Your body has quite successfully grown your baby from 2 cells to a living, thinking, feeling human being....you didn't wake up one morning at 8 weeks and say to yourself 'I need to grow my baby some ears today'....do you really think that your body forgets what to do when it gets to the end of your pregnancy?

- Placenta praevia: This occurs when the placenta is covering the cervical opening. If you went in to labour you and your baby could be in serious trouble. A complete placenta praevia in late pregnancy would automatically mean a caesarean and maybe even a few weeks of bed rest in hospital beforehand. Your caregiver will keep an eye on the position of the placenta during scans. It's quite normal to have a low lying placenta mid-pregnancy, but the placenta usually moves up as the bottom part of the uterus grows. In other words, it will normally self correct — no need for you to do anything. If you are diagnosed with placenta praevia it might be prudent to get a second opinion. One Mum I interviewed recently was preparing for her 4th baby having had three very easy labours and was herself in good health with no problems during her pregnancy. She was diagnosed with placenta praevia and advised that a normal birth would not be possible. Unhappy with this diagnosis Mum got a second opinion at a private hospital and was shocked to learn that she did not have placenta praevia and there were no indications for a caesarean birth. Had this Mum not followed her instincts she would have had major abdominal surgery for no reason. This Mum went on to have her 4th natural birth with no complications.

- Placental abruption is an absolute reason for a caesarean if the placenta begins to come away from your uterine wall causing severe bleeding.

- Prolapsed cord (i.e. when the cord comes out before your baby) in the first stage of labour. (a good reason to avoid routinely break the waters—more on this later)

- Brow presentation.
  If your baby's head isn't well tucked in (chin to chest) and his brow is the presenting part instead of the back of your baby's head a caesarean is likely.

▌ The Debatable Area – When a Caesarean May Not Be Necessary.

Most of Ireland's caesarean sections fall into this category. It is a subjective call by your caregiver and a second opinion might differ considerably.

- Malposition—That means, when your baby is not in a good position i.e. (head down and your baby's chin well tucked in) Depending on the kind of position your baby is in it can make for a more challenging birth or it may require your Doctor/ Midwife thinks outside of the box. If baby is malpositioned sometimes by Mum changing position it can make a difference (stay off the bed!) Also, avoiding breaking the waters routinely is important so the baby can navigate its way through the pelvis with the cushioning of the amniotic fluid.

- Foetal Distress: Most healthy babies tolerate labour exceptionally well but some babies have problems especially if the labour is being induced or accelerated with the chemical hormone Pitocin or if your baby wasn't well to begin with. We'll look at the diagnosis of foetal distress later.

- Dystocia of Labour (failure to progress....or is it failure to wait?) In other words—your time is up.

- You're exhausted: When a mother has been labouring for a long time and is exhausted before the pushing stage.

- Breech for a first baby.

- Nuchal cord (the cord is around your baby's neck). Babies do not get their oxygen through their mouths (windpipe) but through the cord. Nuchal cords are common and occur in around 25%—35% of pregnancies. The research suggests that nuchal cords are "not associated with untoward pregnancy outcomes," "not associated with adverse perinatal outcome," and "do not influence clinical management at delivery."

- Previous 3rd degree perineal injury.
  Although there are no guarantees evidence shows if the second stage is Mother led i.e. no sustained forceful pushing there is less risk to the perineal area. Midwife led coached pushing is an outdated technique still favoured in many Irish units.

▌Breech—Do Not Pass Go—Go Directly to Theatre

Around 4% of babies will be in a breech position at the end of pregnancy. Years ago this wasn't a problem. It used to be quite normal to have a vaginal breech birth in Ireland. My sister and I were both breech and born vaginally. In 2000 a study was published what would forever change how breech babies were born (particularly in hospital). This was known as the Term Breech Trial. The authors of the study concluded unequivocally that caesarean delivery was safer for breech babies. Overnight the caesarean rates grew. But the study was hugely flawed.
Despite a stream of articles discrediting the study it was felt that the conclusions of the study opened the way for more planned caesareans which is what some obstetricians preferred (it's quick and can be planned ahead of time). Supporting a woman giving birth to a breech baby requires skill and patience, a skill that has sadly been lost in most Irish hospitals.

But a breech baby isn't an automatic ticket to theatre. You have options.

Breech vaginal birth—especially if you've given birth normally before—some of the more experienced older consultants are comfortable with breech vaginal birth but many aren't. Undiagnosed breech babies are born in Ireland every year normally—with no complications. Mum progressed quickly and by the time it was obvious that it was a bum rather than a head coming first the baby arrived before the theatre was ready.

ECV (manual turning of your baby by a skilled practitioner and it works 50% of the time). Not all consultants are skilled at ECV but just because yours isn't doesn't mean you can't be referred to one who is. Like any medical intervention it does come with risks but you have a 50% chance of avoiding a caesarean and the risks that come along with surgery. Ask for a referral to your hospital's breech clinic.

Moxa—a traditional Chinese herb burned near the skin by the little toe. Studies show a 70—80% success rate of babies turning.

Hypnosis has also been shown to have a high success rate of around 80%—the deep relaxation of hypnosis allows the uterine muscles to relax completely giving your baby extra room to move.

Caregiver Recommendations

Not all caregivers are created equal. Not all caregivers are familiar with the latest research and evidence and may recommend a caesarean based on a past experience. As a first time Mum trying to determine between an absolute indication backed by medical studies and a vague recommendation for a caesarean can feel like Russian roulette—with very high stakes. A gamble that no mother is willing to take.

Many would find it inconceivable that their caregiver….the Doctor with the lovely bedside manner would perform risky, unnecessary procedures that have been shown time and time again *not* to improve outcomes for Mums and babies. Naturally every Mum believes her caesarean was the one that was absolutely necessary—the alternative is just too painful to consider….but the numbers just don't add up. It's not that these caregivers are being deliberately malicious—but sometimes they're just wrong. In September 2009 the ERSI published a report on the growing numbers of caesarean births in Ireland and suggested that there is a link between private consultant care and the high rates. This point was raised again in November 2009 by the Irish Times.

Following are some of reasons that Mums are given that a caesarean may be the 'best' option.

▌ Are More Doctors Choosing Caesarean Births for Themselves?

What about our caregivers? What kind of births are Obstetricians having? You may have heard of a study where 31% of London Obstetricians who said they would opt for a caesarean birth rather than normal birth (Al-Mufti et al.,1997). However, in countries where the caesarean section rate is less than 20%, such as Norway, Denmark and the Netherlands, similar studies tell a different story – only 1.1–2% of Obstetricians would choose caesarean section for themselves or their partners. These are countries where normal birth is very much supported and birth has not become overly medicalised for women having straight forward normal pregnancies.

▌ Big Baby

Usually announced after several routine 'reassurance scans' and guesstimates of baby's size. Baby is measuring 'large for dates'. Comments of 'we won't let you go over' are common. You'll probably have an early induction (which ups your risk of caesarean by 40%) In your Granny's day before routine ultrasound the Midwife would palpate Nana's tummy and declare—'lovely sized baby'....and Granny would be delighted! Not so long ago 'big' was synonymous with healthy. It meant Granny was growing a healthy baby and in those days with large families, little antenatal care and high levels of poverty—a healthy baby was more likely to survive. A baby that was estimated to be big was considered to good news.

▌ You're Having an IVF Baby

This is an extra special baby and your consultant won't be happy until this baby is in a cot. Considering you have probably done everything in your power to finally get pregnant and keep this baby safe your caregiver now suggests that an early induction/caesarean is the safest option...

Other reasons given to Mums for caesarean surgery that are not based on best practice.

You are over 40

You are over 35

You have small feet/hips

You've had a previous caesarean

You've had 2 previous caesareans
Your last baby was big

You have SPD

Previous tear

Previous penalty points

Christmas

Holy Communion

Opening of Ikea

What Does a Caesarean Really Mean for Your Health?

It's major abdominal surgery—plain and simple. It's the only major surgery performed today where you will be expected to take care of a dependent helpless human being immediately after. Although caesareans have become somewhat 'normal-ised' they do come with a specific set of health risks not just for you but also for you baby.

Risks for Mum include:

- Infection: The uterus or nearby pelvic organs such as the bladder or kidneys can become infected. Wound infections are very common too (can you say MRSA?).

- Increased blood loss: Blood loss on average is about twice as much with caesarean birth as with vaginal birth.

- Growth of adhesions. Over 90% of patients who have had abdominal surgery develop these growths of excess scar tissue. It means your Doctor has to cut through what can look like the thick spiders web that also attaches to other organs. With each surgery these adhesions increase and can affect the functioning of your bowel and your future fertility.

- Hysterectomy or additional surgery to repair the bladder.

- Decreased bowel function: The bowel sometimes slows down for several days after surgery, resulting in distention, bloating and discomfort.

- Respiratory complications: General anaesthesia can sometimes lead to pneumonia (general anaesthesia use is rare for a caesarean).

- Longer hospital stay and recovery time: Five days in the hospital is the common length of stay depending on how busy the unit is, it's usually less than one to three days for a vaginal birth. Readmission to hospital is more common.

- Reactions to anaesthesia: Unexpected responses (such as blood pressure that drops quickly) to anaesthesia or other medications during the surgery.

It is important to keep all of these risks in perspective—you may have a very straight forward caesarean and recover quickly but it's also worth considering the long term impact that a caesarean has on your plans for future pregnancies.

In a 2004 study a team of Scottish Doctors found that women who give birth to their first child by caesarean section may have more trouble getting pregnant again. When compared with Mums who had difficult births ending in vaginal birth, women in the study who had caesarean deliveries said they had more problems getting pregnant after the birth of their first child. Roughly 20% of the caesarean mothers reported difficulty conceiving a second child, compared with 5% of women who had vaginal deliveries.

Naturally the more caesareans you have the more likely you are to experience problems such as:

- ectopic pregnancy: pregnancies that develop outside your uterus or within the scar.

- reduced fertility, due to either less ability to become pregnant again or less desire to do so (especially if you have a difficult labour before your caesarean).
- placenta praevia: the placenta attaches near or over the opening to her cervix.

- placenta accreta: the placenta grows through the lining of the uterus and into or through the muscle of the uterus.
- placental abruption: the placenta detaches from the uterus before the baby is born.

- weakness of the scar on the uterus: the uterine scar gives way during pregnancy or labour.

With a surgical birth, the possible risks to your baby include the following:

- Premature birth: If your due date was not accurately calculated, your baby could be delivered too early and your baby may have to go to special care while you recover in another ward.

- Breathing problems: Babies born by caesarean are more likely to develop breathing problems (normal labour is good for babies!) The passage through the vagina helps to squeeze fluid from your baby's lungs preparing it for life on the outside.

- Low Apgar scores: Babies born by caesarean sometimes have low Apgar scores. The low score can be an effect of the anaesthesia and caesarean birth. A high Apgar score usually means your baby was most likely not in distress to begin with. It can also be due the baby not getting the stimulation he would have gotten in a vaginal birth.

- Foetal injury: The Doctor can accidentally nick the baby while making the incision or have bruising on the face/head from the use of forceps. Sometimes bones are also broken while pulling the baby out. A caesarean can be quite a forceful event on both Mum and baby.

- Less likely to be breastfed. When morphine is the drug of choice in many maternity units it's no wonder breastfeeding is so difficult for first time mothers. There are other options such as Diphene that won't make you drowsy.
- Higher risk of asthma—babies born by caesarean birth are at a higher risk of developing asthma.

- Higher risk of developing Type 1 diabetes.

Of course even a normal vaginal birth also comes with risks. If you have a caesarean you won't experience the temporary perineal pain that is normal for some women after a vaginal birth. You may suffer from incontinence (this is exacerbated by prolonged coached pushing which is no longer recommended) your general health during pregnancy will also impact this. In a difficult vaginal birth some babies can be affected by a nerve injury that affects the shoulder.

The difference is that most of these risks can be reduced or avoided with sensitive Midwifery care and evidence based practices.

Psychological Problems Associated with an Unplanned Caesarean Birth

Mum is less likely to react to her baby positively after being separated. This may not have been the case for you but many women describe feelings of disappointment and confusion when they are finally reunited with their babies if they were separated initially. You may have bonded well with your baby but many Mums don't. You are also at higher risk of depression and risk of PND and PTSD.

Is This My Baby?

A straightforward natural birth involves a complex hormonal cocktail, including oxytocin, the hormone linked to bonding and to feelings of love and trust. Men and women both produce oxytocin during orgasm. Oxytocin is at its highest right after a vaginal birth so if this is bypassed for a caesarean the mother doesn't experience the same hormonal boost of oxytocin for instant bonding.

Dr. Larry Reynolds a Canadian Obstetrician suggests that some women who have had a caesarean section suffer from a kind of post-traumatic stress syndrome especially if they've had a general anesthetic—This is evident when you hear mothers questioning whether they have been given the right baby as you'll have read in the birth stories. Mothers have gone from labouring normally expecting their baby to arrive the way babies have arrived for millions of years and suddenly they are coming around after a GA and handed a child...a child that doesn't feel like theirs. A piece of the process is missing.

In a recently published a study in which six healthy mothers who had caesareans and six who delivered naturally had MRI's taken (images of brain functioning two to four weeks after the births) Researchers measured their brain activity as the women listened to tapes of their babies crying while having their nappies changed. The women who had caesarean births had a slower response time to their baby's crying.

They found that some of the key areas of the brain that regulate sensory processing, empathy, motivation and other emotions were more active in women who had normal vaginal births compared with Mums who'd had caesarean births. Three months later the differences were minimal. But it's not known what may be lost in those critical few weeks. Bonding can happen over a lifetime and you may have not experienced any problems connecting with your baby but many women don't share that same rush of love and wonder if there's something wrong with them.

▌ Failure to Progress—or Failure to Wait?

It's often surprising to first time mothers to find out that the hospital they are attending has strict time limits on how long they will have to give birth. Or if the time limit is mentioned they will assume that there's a good reason for it. Some Mums find this comforting. In theory it sounds great. Who wants to be waiting around in labour for 24 hours when you can have the drive thru option and have your baby in 12 hours or less! We live in a time of instant gratification—instant texts, instant coffee—we've become accustomed to not having to wait for anything anymore. We are also in love with technology and the expected guarantee of safety that the machine that goes 'PING' brings.

Knowing that you are guaranteed to be holding your baby within a specific time frame can be a relief for some. For other Mums this news becomes an added unwanted pressure to an already fearful pregnancy. That's if this information is shared with expectant parents, after all the couple can only make informed decision when they're given all of the facts—and not half of them which is generally the case in antenatal classes that promote managed labours. If you've attended a class like this you've been most likely sold inaccurate, unscientific, biased information wittily presented. Minor details of side effects and risks for you and your baby are not discussed. This is not an antenatal class but an exercise in socialising you in the policies of your unit—policies which you are expected to follow without question—to keep the unit running efficiently. These are essentially 'one size fits all' birth practices. Unless you have expressed some written birth preferences for an individualised care plan for you and your baby you'll just proceed along the production line.

As Henci Goer writes in her acclaimed book 'The Thinking Woman's Guide to a Better Birth'.

Some Obstetricians treat women labouring slowly the way Peter Pan treated the Lost Boys. He expected everyone to adapt to his ideas of the way things should be. If they didn't, Peter saw to it that they did. For example, the boys entered the Neverland underground home through hollow trees. If a boy didn't fit his tree, James Barrie writes, Peter "did something" to the boy. So too with obstetric management. Obstetricians have inflexible ideas of how labour ought to go. If your labour doesn't conform to that pattern, typical Doctors "do something" to you to make you fit. There are, as you may gather, a number of drawbacks to this myopic approach.

Back in the 1960's a package of care for labouring woman was created in the National Maternity Hospital—this philosophy of managing labour to a strict time limit became known as Active Management of Labour. Policies and procedures were devised for high 'turnover' (these days around 8000+ babies are born in NMH). A typically managed birth involves routine amniotomy (breaking the waters) and artificially driving your labour with a synthetic hormone (Pitocin). Both procedures can have serious side effects for Mum and baby and yet continue in our largest maternity unit unchallenged. There is a dangerous assumption that the practice of AML is based on well thought out rigorous scientific studies and research—after all it was created by Obstetricians. But there are no rigorous scientific studies behind AML. In fact the most recent international studies *do not recommend* these routine procedures in a normally progressing labour.

How can this happen? As mentioned earlier there are no National Maternity Guidelines in Ireland unlike most other developed countries. Each hospital decides on it's own policies—and they could be as random as choosing Lotto numbers or based on voodoo because evidence based practices are rare. The closest we have to a maternity watchdog is the volunteer group

AIMS Ireland (Association for the Improvements in Maternity Services).

According to the book on Active Management of Labour active management spares staff the "tedious hours" of waiting until full cervical dilation, and it transforms the "previously haphazard approach" to planning for staffing.

In the book Active Management of Labour penned by Irish Obstetricians Irish Mums have been given their orders—the labouring Mum's job in this scheme of "military efficiency" with a "human face" is to take orders and not to disturb the maternity unit by making "the degrading scenes that occasionally result from the failure of a woman to fulfil her part of the contract.".......this is the philosophy of care at our National Maternity Hospital. Your birth plan is expected to reflect the hospitals staffing plan....not your birth preferences. So you can see why exploring your options can make a difference in how your baby's birth is 'managed'.

Active management also has serious disadvantages. First-time mothers are given oxytocin if they don't steadily progress at the average rate–a rate that is an underestimate. In Cuidiu's consumer guide to Irish maternity services we see that around 35% or more of first-time mothers attending NMH will have their labours chemically driven with synthetic hormones. It is worth pointing out that although NMH has the lowest caesarean rate in Ireland, women giving birth at home or in the care of Midwives have even lower caesarean rates to those at NMH and with better maternal and newborn outcomes so there are other ways to keep birth normal that don't involve chemicals, hooks and forceps. The biggest obstetric intervention is not the forceps...it's the clock.

A new study in the US journal of Obstetrics published in November 2008 suggests that obstetricians can reduce the health risks to mothers and babies by being more flexible with time limits on labour progress. While ACOG in the US already recommends waiting at least two hours with adequate contractions in the setting of no progress in active labour, it is routine practice in many hospitals to proceed with a caesarean for failure to progress before those ACOG criteria have been met. Helen Sandland, an obstetrician in North Caroline resigned in June 2005 after hospital administrators instructed her to increase her caesarean rate (which at the time was 10%). According to Sandland 'c-sections are being done for so called 'failure to progress'. If you haven't progressed in a couple of hours, a caesarean is waiting". Imagine if every woman was expected to have a 28 day menstrual cycle and a period that lasted no more than 3 days....and if you had anything other than this 'standard' which was agreed upon by 3 men in the 1960s then you were considered to have a deficient reproductive system...

FTP or failure to progress or (dystocia as it's commonly known) is responsible for an estimated 1/3 of all caesareans performed in Ireland. The research is clear—a little patience might help avoid several thousand caesareans in Ireland every year. Failure to progress insinuates that the woman's body wasn't performing adequately when in fact she was labouring perfectly normally for her body, her baby and her birth but she was racing the clock. Does the problem really lie with the mother—or with the outdated archaic non scientific routine procedures carried out every day in Irish maternity units? The growing caesarean rate in Ireland has been horribly misdiagnosed—for those mothers who experienced what they were told was a failure to progress was really a failure to wait.

In 2009 an article was published in the US on the impact of reducing the amount of synthetic oxytocin drips. Over 3 years the hospital halved its number of emergency caesarean births. Another significant outcome from this study was a huge decline in emergency vacuum and forceps deliveries. According to Dr. Ventolini who led the study "more and more data is showing us that we are using too much oxytocin—too often".

▌ Time of Day and Intervention Rates

In 2008 the findings of a major study in University College Cork concluded that the time of day or night can influence whether you have a straight forward vaginal birth or a forceps birth.

It seems that the most difficult time for maternity hospitals is after 4.30pm in the evening and overnight until 8.30am, as well as weekends, as they have to cope with reduced staff, tiredness and less experienced Doctors on duty. UCC studied 3,105 births records over a year in one hospital, and found that the majority of babies (67.3%) were born in the evenings, nights and weekends and these were more likely to be delivered by ventouse/vacuum (suction equipment to assist in childbirth).

They found no difference in the rate of caesarean sections carried out during this time, compared to the 8.30am to 4.30pm period.

However, 83% of cases where babies were delivered operatively because of failure to advance in the second stage of labour took place in the evenings and weekends. Is this a case of failure to progress or failure to wait (if you're on call and have been working all night and it's 3am—how patient would you be?)

We'll talk more about this later—specifically how can give you and your baby the best chance of avoiding an unnecessary caesarean.

▌ The Machine that goes 'Ping' and the Rise in Caesarean Births

In the 1960s new technology was developed to listen in to a baby's heart rate during labour. It was thought that if a Mum wore this monitor and her baby was in distress the staff would be alerted and any potential complication would be averted. Electronic Foetal monitoring was originally designed to be used in high risk pregnancies. The original models involved clipping an electrode to the baby's scalp. The company's experts claimed that EFM would save the lives of babies. By 1976 questions about it's accuracy began to come to light and study after study showed a glaring problem—Mothers who were being continuously monitored had a significantly increased rate of caesarean section (30%) and it was not saving any more babies compared to regular listening in by a Midwife. EFM was causing more problems than it was solving but by this time nearly every labour ward in the US had invested heavily in this new technology. There was no going back.

Current evidence recommends that the most appropriate way to monitor your baby (assuming all is well) during labour is intermittent monitoring with a small hand held device called a Sonicaid or with a Pinard (an instrument that looks like a little trumpet). Your Midwife generally listens in every 15—20 minutes and you can be mobile, using the bath, pool or out walking the halls.

But what about a baby that is in distress—surely continuous monitoring would be able to prevent cases of brain damage— wouldn't we be able to tell if a baby was having trouble and save it? Not so. One large study that was carried out in Dublin concluded that babies that were monitored continuously had less seizures—obviously that sounds like it's worth using then. But further analysis showed that these seizures occurred mostly in women that had had their labour speeded up with synthetic oxytocin (Pitocin) and once those figures were adjusted there was no difference in the rates of seizures. Interestingly in the United States 43% of all cases taken against Obstetricians involving brain damaged babies, Pitocin was involved.

One of the problems with using electronic foetal monitoring is not just the machine itself but who is interpreting the information it produces. Guidelines vary between hospitals. It's recommended that if CTG machines are routinely used and there are suspicions of a problem then a sample of blood is taken from your baby's scalp and analysed immediately to determine if your baby is really in trouble or if it's a false alarm….but this is not offered routinely in all Irish maternity units. It depends on whether the Doctor assigned to your care will do it or not—if you are being continuously monitored for any reason and there seems to be a concern for your baby you can request an FBS (foetal blood sampling) and if the Doctor assigned to you or your consultant can't do it—ask for one who can. You do not need to have an epidural for an FBS. Some caregivers prefer Mums to have an epidural for an FBS because it makes their job easier. An epidural impacts your blood pressure and can impact oxygen levels to your baby which can throw off the result. It can be quite uncomfortable but the test can be quickly done in a few minutes. Generally you will be placed on your left side and a cone shaped device is placed into the vagina so the Doctor can see your baby's head. Your baby's head is 'nicked' slightly and a tiny blood sample is taken. The sample is put in a machine that tests your baby's blood to make sure your baby is getting enough oxygen. The entire procedure can take 5—15 minutes to get a definitive answer about your baby's health.

▌ Caesarean Birth and Delayed Cord Clamping

It is becoming more widely accepted that early cord clamping can deprive a newborn of up to half of his intended blood volume at birth so more and more Mums are requesting delayed cord clamping to ensure the healthiest start. Leaving the cord to finish pulsating means your baby's risk of anaemia is significantly reduced and it's especially important for premature babies to protect them from brain bleeds. Leaving your baby attached to it's first 'life support system' for a few extra minutes gives your baby a chance to adapt to using his lungs and reduces cases of respiratory distress (a common issue with caesarean born babies) which usually results in baby going to special care and being separated from Mum and Dad. Early clamping particularly before baby's first breath means blood is sacrificed from other organs (including your baby's heart) to kick-start the lungs. UK paediatrician Peter Dunn recommends that the cord of caesarean babies is left unclamped and that the baby and placenta remain level until the cord stops pulsating in about 8 – 10 minutes. According to Dr. Sarah Buckley your baby could be wrapped and held to your chest for those few moments. Talk to your caregiver about this important option.

Chapter IV

The Journey to VBAC

If you're considering a VBAC (pronounced vee-back) in Ireland there are a couple of things to consider to give yourself and your baby the best chance of having a normal birth.

It's still quite common for Mums to assume that once they've had one caesarean that it's 'game over' and all of their subsequent babies will be born via caesarean. Depending on which maternity unit you are attending support for VBAC is very much hit and miss. VBAC is not routinely offered as the standard plan of care—even though VBAC is known to be safer for you and your baby than a planned caesarean (in a pregnancy without complications). VBAC is also cheaper for the health service..... less infections for Mum = less time in hospital = less re admissions and less time for baby in special care. It makes sense on all levels. Units with very low VBAC rates tend to not have VBAC guidelines in place and any VBAC that happen are what are considered to be 'accidental VBACs' in other words Mum arrived in to the maternity unit in advanced labour and there wasn't a surgeon immediately available to perform the caesarean. Other units differ in their philosophy towards VBAC so their routine standard of care is to encourage VBAC rather than the exception for the majority of low risk Mums. They usually have a VBAC rate of around 60—70%. As you'll see it's all about doing your homework.

Labour is sometimes referred to as an athletic event—to some mothers even a marathon but if you're a VBAC Mum (planning a vaginal birth after a caesarean) you may not even get to start the race because your baby is looking 'big' and a repeat caesarean is recommended or you may not get to finish the race because you'll be disqualified for not completing the race in time. How long should it take? You'll get differing answers depending on which' coaches' you talk to but one thing that is consistent is the supporting research that time limits on labour for VBAC Mums are not necessary as long as Mum and baby are doing ok. Writing down some birth preferences may help you avoid a 'Cinderella' VBAC (it can only happen with specific limitations i.e. before 40 weeks) The same goes for time limits on any labour....there is no evidence that a long labour causes an increase in the risk of scar weakness but there is evidence that an assisted delivery (forceps/vacuum does increase that risk.... again another reason to ask for more time).

There are two distinct levels of care when it comes to having a VBAC in an Irish hospital. There are Mums who challenge the routine offering of a caesarean and insist on being given the best chance at a normal birth. Then there are Mums who don't know that a VBAC is the safest option and are denied informed consent. These Mums are misled into believing a planned caesarean is in their best interest.

VBAC is often a very lonely road for Irish Mums especially in a VBAC 'shy' unit compared to the UK's attitude to VBAC. You'll hear that you could die if you insist on trying for VBAC or worse still that your baby could die. According to birth expert Henci Goer no study in the VBAC literature recorded a maternal death attributable to VBAC.
Even still you may be inclined to assume that a planned caesarean is the way to go but ironically the risk of maternal death is twice that of a vaginal birth. VBAC is associated with a lower risk of complications for both Mum and baby than a repeat caesarean.

Of course there may be an occasion when VBAC is not possible but as long as you feel you are part of the decision making process you can still have a very positive birth experience.

A good chance at VBAC in Ireland takes work—how much do you want it? What are you willing to do to have a normal birth? Don't get me wrong this is not about putting you or your baby's health at risk this is not about 'VBAC at any cost'.... but you'll have to take some emotional risks with your self esteem and your confidence and move out of your comfort zone by questioning policies and practices so you know right from the beginning that you, your hospital and caregivers are on the same page.

▐ Understanding the Risks

According to Canadian obstetrician Andrew Kotaska we live in a culture of 'risk magnification'. We tend to focus on the small unlikely risk rather than the bigger picture that with appropriate care in all likelihood everything will go perfectly well. Midwives tend to focus on best case scenario whereas Obstetricians focus on worst case – simply because Midwives see far more normality than Obstetricians.

You'll probably have some statistics thrown at you—the most frequently referenced statistic is that your risk of scar separation is 0.5% or 5 in 1000 or 1 in 200. Look at it from another perspective—you have a 99.95% chance of having a normal birth. These are very good odds! If you choose a repeat caesarean you have a 99.8% chance of not having a scar separation (it's still a risk even in a caesarean birth) and a 100% chance of major surgery and all of the complications that come along with a planned caesarean.

From 1976-2005, 19 peer-reviewed studies on uterine rupture reported 1654 cases of uterine rupture among 2,504,456 pregnant Mums, the overall rupture rate was 1 in 1514 pregnancies (0.07%).

But for a lot of Mums 1 in 200/ 5 in 1000+ seems like a very high risk and they assume that this means they have a 1 in 200 chance of losing their baby or their own life but this just isn't the case. True uterine rupture is very rare.

Let's look at that 'R' word (rupture)...according to Enkin et al a true scar separation is rare and although often considered to be the most common cause of uterine rupture, previous caesarean section is a factor in less than HALF the reported cases'. So in fact more than half of the women who have problems with a tear in the uterus have never even had a caesarean. One thing that rarely comes up in discussions in a VBAC 'shy' maternity unit is the increased risk for you and your baby with a planned caesarean. A planned caesarean although gives the illusion of safety is the less healthy option in a normal pregnancy for you and your baby. A study published by the WHO in Jan 2010 once again demonstrated that Mums and babies are at increased risk of health problems.

Some consultants can be quite VBAC shy—this usually shows itself around the 38 week when there's talk of baby's size and only 'allowing' you to go to a certain date before a caesarean is on the cards. With appropriate care, 70 to 85% of women who have an opportunity for a VBAC will have an uncomplicated normal birth that is well supported by research. In Jennifer Block's controversial book 'Pushed' Dr. Mark Landon a well known VBAC supporter claims that Mums are not getting accurate information on which to base a decision and as a Doctor he confirmed that he could talk most Mums into either option if that was what he wanted to do. While researching this book I found that several Irish units have VBAC rates of 60 – 70% but shockingly some units rates are less than 5%. Not all maternity units were willing to provide their statistics.

Recently the British Journal of Obstetrics published a very positive study by Dr Turner at the Coombe with some really encouraging results for Irish Mums who are considering VBAC.

Out of 4021 women 78% had a successful VBAC. There were 9 cases of scar separation—6 of the 9 were induced or had oxytocin during the labour. According to Dr Turner even when the scar separated, major complications for mother or baby were few. Sadly even with this encouraging research VBAC rates are going down in the Coombe from 90% in 1986 to 49% in 2006—why? Because of the fear of scar weakness. **The risk to your baby from the very low incidence of scar separation (less than 1%) is much less than the risk to your baby from respiratory distress (wet lungs) as a result of a planned caesarean (around 3%).**

▌ Uterine Rupture / Scar Separation

There's no doubt that a *true* UR can be catastrophic—thankfully these are extremely rare. There are different types of uterine rupture from complete to incomplete and most studies of VBAC did not differentiate between them which really clouds the issue.

Incomplete Uterine Rupture

This is categorised in a number of ways:
- uterine window
- partial scar dehiscence
- occult uterine rupture
- silent rupture

In the vast majority of the above scenarios the uterus heals perfectly well, and it does not result in a repeat caesarean and can sometimes go undetected. Mum and baby experience no problems from these kinds of rupture.

The main reason for these 'asymptomatic' ruptures (meaning no symptoms) being discovered is the former practice of uterine exploration by the surgeon. The Obstetrician would explore your uterus with his hands after your baby was born to look for any signs of separation. You would imagine at a significant amount of pain and discomfort for the woman. This is a practice now acknowledged by most Obstetricians as being unnecessary and not best practice.

The other cases where a uterine dehiscence (weakness) may be discovered is at the time of a repeat caesarean. You may have heard stories of Mums being told that that the scar was very thin or about to rupture or her uterus was 'see through'. This is usually only a case of dehiscence and comments such as this do not reflect evidence based medicine.

▓ Factors that are Thought to Impact Scar Strength

There are a few factors to consider in terms of VBAC.

- Type of scar
- Labour induction
- Type of uterine rupture

VBACs have historically gotten a bad rap as the old style classical incision is weaker. Induction can overstimulate the uterus and makes a rupture more likely—even in a uterus *without* a previous caesarean. It's hard to differentiate in the early studies whether a scar problem is really an issue or if it's a uterine dehiscence (a 'dehiscence' is where the scar starts to undo, but only by a small amount; neither Mum nor baby are affected. These are often called 'asymptomatic' scar separations as no symptoms are shown by Mum or baby.

True uterine scar separation is generally distinguished from asymptomatic (no signs of a problem) scar separation (dehiscence) by the need for emergency surgery, although some reports combine these separate processes which just confuses everything! The rate of true uterine rupture with one prior low-transverse scar has been reported in the US to be between 0.2 and 1.5 percent (one of 67 to 500 women). Other studies involving more than 130,000 women rates that average 0.6 percent (approximately one of every 170 women). (Toppenberg 2002). True uterine scar separation is *symptomatic*, which means that the mother begins to loose blood which affects her blood pressure, and restricts blood to the baby. She may or may not feel pain when this is happening.

So, when you hear horror stories of an exploding uterus it's important to ask what type of scar, was Mum's labour induced or accelerated in some way – did she have an assisted delivery? It is important to have all of the information of any contributing factors.

If you're having a hard time getting past the issues around potential scar problems there are a couple things to consider when looking at scar separation. Even if you schedule a planned caesarean there is still a risk of scar separation (albeit a lower one). While the rates of scar separation among women who opt for a repeat caesarean are lower, you have to take into account the additional risks associated with major abdominal surgery. Take your time and decide which option you feel most comfortable with.

'A Guide to Effective Care in Pregnancy and Childbirth', which is a well-respected summary of evidence-based maternity practice, says "To put these rates into perspective, the probability of requiring an emergency caesarean section for acute other conditions (foetal distress, cord prolapse, or antepartum haemorrhage) in any woman giving birth, is approximately 2.7%, or up to 30 times as high as the risk of uterine rupture with a planned vaginal birth after caesarean".

A true scar separation is very rare and the incidence of this happening is comparable to other obstetrical emergencies such as placental abruption which has a worldwide rate of 1%.

As Obstetrician Mona Lydon-Rochelle said at the US National Institute of Health's VBAC conference in March 2010, "There is a major misperception that choosing VBAC is extremely risky". Obstetrician George Macones stated in terms of VBAC, "Your risk is really, really quite low." Additionally, the risk of infant death during a VBAC attempt is "similar to the risk" of infant death during the birth of a first time mom (Smith, 2002).

If you've had a previous caesarean, your risk of needing emergency caesarean in future rises from around 2.7% to around 3.2%. **Even taking higher figures for uterine scar separation, you are still more than five times more likely to need an emergency caesarean for other reasons, than for uterine rupture.**

A 2006 Israeli study suggests a non induced, non accelerated and drug free labour is the safest form of VBAC. Of the 800+ Mums who planned a VBAC—80% had one. One scar separation occurred hours after the baby was born.

▌ I Haven't Laboured Before—What Are My Odds Of Having A VBAC.

The reason for your last caesarean is important. If you had an elective caesarean for a breech baby or placenta praevia (so you didn't labour yourself the last time) you have as good a chance at a normal birth as a first time Mum. If you had a caesarean because of a problem that you now have again then VBAC wouldn't be recommended. Usually there is no reason to expect that the same problem will occur again. in the past, particularly if it was a VBAC. According to the RCOG 2007 & 2008—VBAC success is between 72% and 76% if you've had one previous caesarean.

If you've given birth vaginally to at least one baby in the past then the VBAC rates are between 87 per cent and 90%.

▌ When Can I Start Trying for Another Baby

This is such a personal decision but there are several studies that can help you make the best decision for you and may increase your chances of a vaginal birth. Unfortunately some of the studies included the use of prostaglandins to induce a VBAC labour which of course we know is a big no no so it's difficult to ascertain which studies are in fact quality studies! The scar in the uterus is thought to be healed by 6 months. Overall the findings were that the shorter the interval between pregnancies the higher the risk of scar problems. Most studies recommend not having an EDD less than 18 months since your last surgery. If you do find yourself becoming pregnant sooner than that it will be critical to discuss avoiding chemical induction with your caregiver to give yourself the best chance at VBAC.

▌ My Last Baby was Big—Will Another Big Baby Affect My Chances of VBAC?

We know that scans are not an accurate measure of a baby's size. The general consensus from the most recent studies is that VBAC odds are better in a baby weighing less than 9lbs (4000g). But there are always exceptions. No one knows exactly how much your baby will weigh until after the birth. According to the UK Government's CESDI (Confidential Enquiry into Stillbirths & Deaths in Infancy) report "the inaccuracy of ultrasound estimates have been well documented. Indeed, it is possible that estimating fetal weight by late ultrasound may do more harm than good by increasing intervention rates". There is a great UK site that is all about 'big babies' and information on larger VBAC babies—I've included the link in the resource section at the back of the book.

▌ The Bottom Line

If you do not have a compelling medical reason for a caesarean, having a VBAC rather than a repeat caesarean section is likely to be:

> Far safer for you and your baby in this pregnancy and in any future pregnancies.

In fact, looking at all the reproductive risks of a planned caesarean: fertility challenges, increased risk of ectopic pregnancy, stillbirth, preterm labour, small for gestational age, malformation, central nervous system injury, it becomes clear that the scarred uterus and the presence of surgical adhesions make a much less hospitable environment for nurturing future babies." from Elective Caesarean Surgery Versus Planned Vaginal Birth: What Are the Consequences published by Lamaze International.

▌ I'm Planning a VBAC—What Happens if I Go Over?

Studies have shown that a VBAC Mum who gives birth before 40 weeks or after 40 weeks have similar outcomes (approx 65—73% successful VBACs). In the 2006 Israeli study Mums were only induced at 42 weeks and prostaglandins (gel/pessaries) were not used. As many Irish Mums find as their EDD approaches their caregiver out of the blue announces that 'we won't let you go over—if you haven't gone into labour by X we'll get you in for another section'. Out comes the diary to schedule you in for your caesarean on which ever day your Doctor does his planned sections.

Sometimes induction is suggested. When it comes to induction of labour after a previous caesarean two words sum it up perfectly—**not recommended**. Does it happen? Yes. Mums with a prior caesarean who are induced have a 33-75% risk of having another caesarean. Chemical induction or augmentation (speeding up of your labour) is known to increase the risk of scar problems during birth. A scarred uterus needs TLC and patience. In a recent birth story I received from a mother approaching her 'guess date' prostaglandin gel was suggested if she went 'over'—thankfully Mum had done her research and was able to confidently discuss with her Doctor the risks of this form of induction for a VBAC Mum.

One Mum attending a Dublin maternity unit enquired about the option of going past 14 days if she and her baby were well. Her caregiver implied that at that point the hospital would no longer be considering her choices but the health of the baby under the Irish Constitution.....we can only guess at what that might mean.....

Pregnancy should be a time of relaxed anticipation.... Mothers should not have to spend their pregnancies pouring over research papers becoming mini Obstetricians to ensure they are getting the most up to date safest evidence based care available.

In 2005, another study concluded "in women with previous caesarean section and no vaginal deliveries, induction of labour carries a relatively high risk of uterine rupture/dehiscence despite all precautions" Another study found that inducing or accelerating/augmenting a Mum's labour doubled the cases of scar separation.

As long as you and your baby are fine, there is no reason to induce simply because you have gone over your guess date.
Ask your caregiver for the studies that show going past your EDD is a problem and ask for more time.

▌ Is There Any Way to Estimate My Risk of Having a Scar Separation?

In 2005 a group of Obstetricians in the Scotland developed a model to predict the risk of emergency caesarean section among Mums who wanted a VBAC and to determine whether Mums at increased risk of caesarean section were also at increased risk of having their scar separate during the birth.

They split the women into two groups; using one group, they developed a way of predicting the outcome (whether or not the women were going to need an emergency caesarean section) by looking at various risk factors including mother's age, height, sex of baby, gestation, and whether and how the birth was induced. Then, using the second group of women, they tested the model they had developed. They discovered that they could identify half of the women as being at high or low risk of needing emergency caesarean section, with the remainder being at intermediate risk. Some of the factors that increased the risk were older maternal age, smaller height, male sex of baby, labour induced by prostaglandin, not having had a previous vaginal birth, and later birth. They also found that the risk of having a scar separation went up as the risk of emergency caesarean section went up.

▐ VBAC—Is it Worth the Trouble?

Only you can decide. If you've had a previous difficult labour that ended in a caesarean it's understandable why a calm, controlled caesarean seems like the obvious choice next time around. Imagine calmly and excitedly walking to theatre, your spinal block is administered and within a few minutes you hear the lusty cry of your new baby. Sounds perfect! Other than lack of hospital/caregiver support the next biggest obstacle faced by a Mum considering VBAC is fear. A previous negative experience of birth contributes most to the fear of future births and is one of the most common reasons that Mums request a planned caesarean. Psychologists in Scandinavia have developed very effective strategies for reducing the *perceived* need for a caesarean by debriefing sessions and psychological exercises for Mums. Swedish and Finnish reports suggest that more than half of Mums withdraw their request for a planned caesarean after being able to discuss their anxieties and fears and debrief a traumatic experience. Irish Mums generally don't get a chance to debrief a traumatic birth experience unless you actively pursue it yourself through the complaints process.

After experiencing a debriefing with a psychologist according to Nerum (2006) 86% of Mums changed their original request for caesarean section and decided to go for VBAC. Follow-up surveys confirmed that the Mums were very satisfied with their decision to change their request even if they didn't have a VBAC due to a complication in the end.

If you're in two minds about what's the best decision for you there are a couple of things to consider. First off second pregnancies are rarely the same and it's very unlikely that you would be induced for VBAC.

If you're unsure about VBAC a debriefing can be very helpful. It might be worth reviewing your hospital notes with and see if your first caesarean could have been avoided. Sometimes they can't be. I've worked with Mums who have had previous caesareans because of long difficult inductions (simply because it was policy to induce at x days over). At the time they were led to believe that their baby was too big/Mum was too small/wrong star sign etc....and Mum goes on to give birth to an even bigger baby normally 2 years later. Other Mums are told they have 'low' fluid only to find out their fluid levels were in fact normal for that stage of pregnancy. A caesarean puts a woman's entire reproductive life, including subsequent pregnancies, at higher risk of having problems. It's worth considering the bigger picture especially if you are planning to have more children. Request a meeting with a staff member or contact AIMS and they can recommend someone to debrief your notes with you.

▌ Which Hospital Has the Best VBAC Rate?

In researching my book I contacted every maternity unit in Ireland by phone and email. I received no response from over half of our maternity units. Under these circumstances no news is not good news. Of those hospitals who did chose to provide their information the VBAC rates varied considerably. One regional hospital who did provide their statistics has a VBAC rate of less than 5% compared to some units which have an impressive rate of 60 – 70%. Hospitals with no written VBAC clinical guidelines in place tend to have the most negative attitudes towards VBAC which translates into the lowest rates.

▌ How Can I Find Out the Rate of My Local Hospital?

Before you decide which hospital to attend (or whether home-birth might be for you) write to the Director of Midwifery or Head of Obstetrics in the maternity unit you're considering and request their VBAC rate and whether they have written guidelines for VBAC. Finding the most supportive caregiver for VBAC is generally word of mouth – talk to other VBAC Mums.

CHAPTER V

VBAC BIRTH STORIES

Reasons Why Mums Choose VBAC

Siobhan says—"I had a section on my first labour due to failure to progress. The phrase stuck in my head and I began to wonder did this mean that I was not capable of giving birth—something I assumed my body was made to do. The feeling that I had missed out on giving birth to my child grew inside of me and long before I fell pregnant with my second child I had decided that this was the route I wanted go down. I personally found the medical staff in Waterford Regional fantastic in supporting my choice. Although I had another section (a crash section in the end), I wouldn't change my decision.

I still feel like I have missed out on a wonderful experience— giving birth. I split hairs about this phrase as I don't believe that I technically gave birth to my children—the surgeon did. However, my husband and I gave life to them and they are healthy and beautiful. This definitely overshadows any sense of loss".

I chose VBAC for quite a few reasons. I wanted a faster recovery than I had with my first daughter particularly because I now have to go home to a three year old who obviously needs a fair amount of attention. I really didn't want to go through all the operative risks again—all the pain killers, not being able to walk, post op infections etc. The main reason though was because when I had my emergency caesarean with my first daughter I just felt totally interfered with, ignored by staff and had my personal space invaded in a very different way than I'd felt before. I wanted the experience to be private for my husband and I and I wanted to feel everything for myself and the section had left me feeling just numb. I really wanted something natural and primitive, not clinical with every medical student under the sun watching!

Sadly I didn't get my VBAC but still managed to have a positive experience.

I haven't had baby number two yet but I had an emergency c section six months ago and I am determined to have VBAC next time. I have many reasons for this. I found the section very difficult to recover from and it also meant I was unable to fulfil some of my birth plans. I had hoped the cord could be left in tact until it had finished pulsating and this did not happen, I also had wanted to put baby to the breast as soon as he was born and instead we were separated for two hours. I had also wanted to avoid epidural and could not do this. I had all of these things in my birth plan as I felt these would be best for baby. The recovery after the section physically has been difficult and slow and emotionally I found it very hard to come to terms with not delivering the baby myself. These are some of the many reasons I would be determined to have a VBAC.

I had an emergency section on my first and really wanted a VBAC on my second. I had a successful VBAC last May. There were a lot of reasons why I wanted a VBAC. I found the recovery on the section very hard, also was separated from baby for 4 hours (I had to go to recovery until feeling came back in my legs) which I found awful and also having a toddler at home I knew if I had a section I wouldn't be able to lift him which I knew would be hard on him trying to explain that mammy couldn't pick him up. I also wanted to experience a natural delivery as I felt I missed out on some of the bonding experience with the section. I am so glad now that I experienced a natural delivery—it was definitely a much better experience than section,

I had emergency section on my first son and hope to have VBAC on this baby. I have no regrets or disappointment over having had a section on my little boy, it was a case that my son would not survive a normal delivery and I'm just glad I have him here to trash my house daily! I would like to have a VBAC this time simply for the fact I don't want to have to spend as long in hospital after section and I want to be able to hold my new baby and my son without worrying about stitches.

I understand some women feel that they have been robbed of a precious moment, I didn't have my son with me for 2 hours after delivery and my heart and body ached for him, so I appreciate that women feel the need for this process or moment in labour. I do feel looking back on my stay in hospital that it was probably the best thing that could have happened to me. We were nearly 2 weeks in hospital after section and it was just me and my son, what better way to get to know your baby or learn your new trade as a Mammy! I have stopped researching VBACs at the moment. I'm reading too much negative information and trying to keep positive, I won't be devastated if I have section in the end but I am a very stubborn person and once an idea is in my head I will do whatever it is! My consultant said as she was taking my son out that just because one child is section it does not mean I can't go on to have a "normal" birth. I thought that was a positive little plant at the back of my mind at a special moment! Glad she said it; it keeps me going when I get a doubt. I just want a healthy situation for this next baby to arrive in and am hoping VBAC is that.

I had an emergency caesarean on my daughter (failure to induce) she was very high and wasn't moving down after 9 hours of attempted induction. I was so determined to have a VBAC, my reasons being I felt I was robbed of the birth experience, I didn't feel I gave birth to my daughter. I also found the recovery from the section very difficult and as my daughter was only going to be 21 months when my son was born I knew having another section was going to be worse.

I spent hours online researching VBACs and speaking to other Mums about successful and unsuccessful VBACs to try and get more information on how to succeed.

At 41 weeks my son was very high (same as my daughter). I was examined in the hospital to see if I was suitable for induction, we decided in the end to go for a section as I wasn't favourable and I didn't feel that waiting another week would make any difference.

As I was in the hospital waiting for the section (12 hours waiting) I went into labour, I was having contractions for hours before I told anyone and from when I was examined it was another 2 hours before I was brought down for the section and in all this time my son still had not budged.

I thought I would be more disappointed at having another section but funnily enough it didn't bother me, I felt I had given it my best shot and there must have been a reason why both babies would not move down. The recovery was also much better than I expected and much easier than with my daughter. I do credit using hypnosis for birth for my calm acceptance of the situation.

I have no regrets about my emergency caesarean because my son was in serious trouble and I have no doubt in my mind that it was the right thing to do at the time. His cord was compressed and we had to have a general anesthetic because the situation was so acute. However my consultant said I'd have a 3 in 4 chance of a VBAC next time, if I go into labour on my own and I would love it—I hated the section recovery period and feel it seriously compromised my ability to exclusively breastfeed amongst other things. So I will prepare for a vaginal birth, same as last time, and see how things go.

My daughter was born suddenly by section after a routine antenatal appointment at 39+4 revealed she was breech (having been head down previous week). I felt very disappointed that I had not experienced a normal delivery but events transpired against me with regards to timing, fluids being low etc.

I was determined on my son to go for a VBAC; no other option would do and was given a 70-80% chance of success. I really wanted to get the normal delivery experience—contractions, pushing baby out, the sense of achievement—all the things I missed out on first time around as well as not having to recover from major surgery when I had a toddler at home.

In hindsight I did not do as much research as I should have or could have and just thought it would either happen or not....obstetrician had said no induction—so I would have to go into labour myself and he would only allow me to go 1 week overdue and would section me if nothing had happened. I hadn't planned for the grey area that occurred....my waters broke at 40+2 so I assumed I would get my VBAC but labour didn't progress, contractions were sporadic and after 26 hours they recommended another section.

I was definitely not prepared for the disappointment at not getting it although I have come to terms with it now. If I ever get pregnant again I will be researching the possibility of VBA2C (not that they will let me) but I will be far more prepared!

I felt I had nothing to lose by going for a VBAC. Although my previous consultant had recommended an elective section on my first for suspected macrosomia (big baby), I had a spontaneous labour and the reason for the section in the end was failure to dilate with Grade III meconium in the fluid, increasing maternal blood pressure and signs of foetal distress.

I was given a 70% chance of a successful VBAC, assuming spontaneous labour again, despite my son also measuring above the 95%ile at 40 weeks and he was born a week later.

However, on my third pregnancy, I opted for an elective section when I was 40w4d as I was by then confined to bed with SPD and was afraid of doing serious, permanent damage to my pelvis should I need to use either McRoberts or Gaskin manoeuvres again (my son had a mild shoulder dystocia during the second stage).

Aoife and Brian Prepare for their VBAC

Background
I was hoping not to go 15 days overdue as I had with my first son which ended in an emergency section, something I never thought would happen to me and something I was totally unprepared for. I don't know how you prepare for a section but maybe afterwards if someone has the time to explain to you that you may feel very upset and that is normal. I did not realise until months later that the way I felt is the way many woman feel.

My VBAC labour

I was due November 27th and on the morning of November 21st I felt like I was going to get my period. It was such a mild feeling but I thought that something might happen.
I got my first surge when I got up from a nap at about 4 o'clock but things did not kick off properly until 4.30 and once it

started it was intense from the very beginning. I got into the bath almost straight away and stayed there until we left for the hospital.

Brian counted through each surge and that is what got me through my labour at home. Brian said the contractions were 1-2 minutes apart always from when he arrived at 4.30. By 6 o'clock I knew things were going faster than I would have expected. I was sleeping between each contraction even though they were really intense. We left the house around seven, it took ages to get ready as I needed my other half with me for each contraction [every 1-2 minutes] so packing the car and getting dressed took for ever. He was literally running about doing everything in between each surge and then racing back to count me through.

I got in the car and bent over a beanbag and some pillows across the back seat. We left the house at about 7. I felt my waters go in the car before we even pulled out. It was a couple of slow trickles.

Once we got down the driveway I was insisting we stop for the contractions, the bumps were a nightmare and I could barely stay on the seat (we live in the countryside on back roads). We ended up driving for one minute and then stopping, the contractions were on top of each other. The contractions were a nightmare once we were in the car, probably because my waters were gone. I could feel my bones moving and feel myself opening. We were making terrible progress in terms of getting there because of all the stopping. At a certain point everything changed and I felt the baby was coming. I told my husband to call an ambulance and to stop. I couldn't handle the car and felt the baby was going to come as my body was sort of convulsing and I could feel it open up and I felt it was pushing something out as it sort of convulsed.

We met the ambulance after a couple of minutes. The ambulance men were lovely. I felt like I could barely move from the car, I eventually crawled through the car on all fours onto their stretcher. Once in the ambulance they tried to decide what to do—whether to stay and deliver the baby or make a move for the hospital. They said they felt they should make it as it was only 5 minutes away. They journey was awful I was on all fours and had my eyes closed from when I got into the ambulance until we got to the labour ward. There were two Midwives there in the room with my file when we arrived. It was just gone eight o'clock. One nurse tried to help me take the gas and air I think I just bit the mouthpiece instead of breathing it in the other nurse was trying to listen for the baby's heartbeat. I was lying on my side/front. I could not move at all.

It took a little while to find the heart beat and the nurses were starting to get really worried. Brian said it was really low down compared to where they were looking. He said they were looking on my tummy and when they found it it seemed to be really low down in my pelvis area. The heartbeat was perfect and strong.

After about 20 minutes of being there and the Midwives talking to me I was in a better state. They did a great job in helping me get back my focus which I did thankfully. They even read my detailed birth plan. It's worth doing a plan or having one especially if you arrive in and are not in a position to go through your wishes.

The Midwife asked could she examine me to see, I found it hard to be still she said the baby was just there but there might be some lip stopping it coming down fully, she was not sure. The consultant checked and moved it during a contraction.

Within a minute they said the baby was there but they had been saying this since I arrived so I didn't realise the baby was on the way out. They said to push if I had the urge and I didn't realise it but during each contraction that is what was happening my body convulsing [as I call] it was the baby moving down.

I was sitting up and felt comfortable in this position. I thought I would prefer to stand but it was too hard for me to move much. I think it took me about 2 -3 contractions to work with my body and realise that when my body convulsed I was actually pushing. A new Midwife came in and the other two were still there, it was probably close to changeover time. The new Midwife said ok push for this contraction whenever it comes. I did push but my body pushed really strongly too. The Midwife shouted to stop pushing.

I think he came out in one shot, they told me to look down and he was there—all of him, I thought I was going to be pushing for a while so could not believe it was all over just like that! He looked huge to me, he was calm, his eyes were open and he had his hands together and was looking around. I really could not believe that he was here and it was over already. He was born at 8.50pm—45 minutes after we arrived.

The consultant was in the room for the delivery but mostly he stayed in the background. He interjected at one point and told me I would be hoarse or loose my voice if I didn't do something differently. He tried to explain what to do. I didn't really realise he was in the room for the delivery.

I had asked for a natural 3rd stage which I got. It felt uncomfortable when the placenta came out but fine not sore at all. However they were worried I was bleeding. The Midwife and the consultant kept pushing my tummy and I could feel all the blood come out. I started breastfeeding and they said that would help but they still seemed to be worried about the bleeding I told them I had no problem with the injection and the consultant said it would probably be fine but they both seemed relieved when I said I would have it.

I had asked for the cord to be left pulsate and when it had the Midwife asked Brian did he want to cut the cord, he didn't and I was in too much shock [happy shock] to do it! The consultant had to give me stitches, I got 5-6 stitches. I don't know if it could have been avoided I don't think they were expecting him to shoot out.

Babs was wrapped in a blanket or two and left with us. The lights were turned down and we were left alone I was breast-feeding him and he knew what to do. The Midwife wanted us to have some nice time which we did. She made sure we had everything we needed and said she was next door and left us to ourselves.

We were left in the labour room until 12. Brian went and got a taxi to our car ad he came back to the labour ward with the bags and the Midwife ordered us both tea and toast. He weighed 8lbs 11oz. The outfit I brought for him to wear was too short. He is very long. He fed for ages.

How we Prepared for our VBAC

I would have spent ages on the internet reading about VBACs and doing my own research about methods of induction, I probably read up at least 2-3 hours a week on the internet, almost to the point of obsession.

I also read Tracy Donegan's Better Birth Book, Ina May Gaskins book and Ricki Lake's book.

I did the home Gentlebirth VBAC course. I found the Gentlebirthing wonderful during my pregnancy. I found it made me calm and let me feel confident about a VBAC. I did the home course and if we have another baby we will hopefully do the weekend course. During the labour I never worried once about having a section. Once I got the feeling I was going to go into labour I believed it was going to happen the way I had hoped.

For anyone planning a VBAC I think the key areas are to have a supportive person with you who is as well informed as you are. Brian was great I felt his support and desire for me to have a VBAC hugely. He had read what I asked him to read. He had developed opinions on various aspects of childbirth which were similar to mine and he knew what I wanted. He never once suggested going to the hospital even though he said he felt things were happening quickly. He said he just wanted to try and have me relaxed so he just tried to do what I wanted/needed. He told me to relax my jaw during the contractions and at the very end when baby came out. I had asked him to remind me to do all these random things…as we do! He was so thrilled for me, just before the baby came he said with tears in his eyes—'oh Aoife you are going to have the natural birth you wanted.' He's the best.

I also found my consultant very positive towards having a VBAC. He always felt if I went in to labour myself there would be no problems and he never spoke about a section so I never felt pressure. When I went overdue on my first he agreed to support me going 17 days overdue provided I came in daily for monitoring so I feel he judges the situation and does not have 'rules'. I felt his delight/warmth for me having gotten what I hoped for. I went to 8 and a half centimetres on my first and the cons always said that would really be in my favour—he felt I had an 80% chance of a VBAC but I put all statistics out of my head as I could only consider a 100% chance. I went private as I felt the care was good first time around. I did consider going public, but I felt the best decision for me was to go private.

Aoife and Brian's Reasons for Choosing a VBAC

I never considered anything else and it became so important to me even before I was pregnant. I read up a lot about VBACs ^ter I had my first son and then decided to leave the matter ` until I was pregnant. I decided to wait a while to have baby. One reason was to allow my body heal from the ^elt it made sense for me to wait and allow the most ^le.

I don't know why it was so important. I have meet people who never minded having a section. I always wanted a large family and I knew that while other people have had five sections I never would. I think it takes a huge toll on your body. I wanted to have a family of five and I knew if I had a section on my second birth I would probably stop at that. The idea that another section would limit or alter my family forever seemed like a threat in the background.

I also never had surgery and not being prepared was awful. I don't think anyone can be prepared. I remember my body shaking after the op. I was definitely in shock for a while. Dealing with masses of visitors while trying to learn how to breastfeed, recover from a major operation and mind a new unsettled baby was horrendous. So I wanted to avoid being in that position.

I live in the middle of nowhere which I love. However not being able to drive with a new baby was awful. I felt stuck. I couldn't leave the house if I wanted so I had to put up with all the visitors (I am so ungrateful, wouldn't it be worse to be alone).

I felt I missed out on something in a way. I had gone through a long labour so I knew how it felt. I knew it was hard work..... but I felt I was not part of the group of woman who have a normal labour. I look after myself, I exercise and have a healthy diet and I am a vegetarian. I like all things natural, gentle as nature meant them and certainly there is little natural about having a section.

Having had a natural birth I cannot believe the difference. I never had a tearful moment. No baby blues at all. I felt so happy for myself as I felt SO GOOD! It's fantastic. It also made coming home to a two year old a lot easier as I could pick him up for cuddles.

Our Birth Preferences
Our Wishes for Childbirth—Aoife & Brian

Due Date: 11/27/2009

18/10/2009

To whom it may concern, We are looking forward to the birth of our second child at Wexford General. We are hoping and planning for a vaginal birth and would appreciate any support in achieving this. I have been practising Gentlebirthing for the last couple of months. We have prepared a 'wishlist' of our preferences in relation to pain relief and procedures. We understand things may change during labour and we may need to revise this. Please keep us informed as to our best options at all times.

Thank you for your help,

Labour
• I would like to be free to walk around and move during labour.
• I would prefer to keep the number of vaginal exams to a minimum, particularly if my waters have ruptured.
• I do not wish to have continuous fetal monitoring, I would like to be monitored on arrival and then intermittently after this.
• I do not want to have the amniotic membrane ruptured.
• I do not want to have oxytocin or anything similar.
• I would like the environment to be kept as quiet as possible.
• I would like the lights in the room to be kept low during my labour [if this is possible?].
• I would prefer not to have an episiotomy unless absolutely required for the baby's safety.
• I am hoping to protect the perineum. I have been practising by squatting, doing Kegel exercises and perineal massage.
• I would appreciate guidance in when to push and when to stop pushing so the perineum can stretch.

Pain Medication

• I do not want Pethidine and/or sleeping tablets, both of these made me feel awful the last time.

• I would like to try and have as a natural birth as possible.

• I do not want to have an epidural. If I ask for one please remind me that I wanted to try and avoid an epidural to improve my chances of having a vaginal birth. If I really insist please make me wait until after I am 5cm.

• I found the gas and air good the last time so if I am looking for pain relief this would be my preference.

Immediately After Delivery

• I would love to have the baby placed on my stomach/chest immediately after delivery.

• I would like to breastfeed the baby soon after delivery.

• I would prefer that the umbilical cord stop pulsating before it is cut.

• Ideally if I have had a natural labour/birth I do not want an injection after the delivery to aid in expelling the placenta.

Caesarean

• If I have to have a section please show me my baby and let me hold my baby immediately after delivery, this is very important to me.

• Brian will stay with the baby at all times—please wrap the baby in blankets & sheets but do not dress him/her.

Please get me back to the ward asap so I can be with my baby and breastfeed my baby

I had my first c-section in 2002 when my baby went into distress after an induction—I was 40+12. I had 2 prostin gels and several hours after my second my waters were broken (with my permission) as the trace was showing distress. Grade 3 meconium was found and I was rushed to theatre for an emergency section.

I opted for VBAC on my next pregnancy for a few reasons:

1) I felt it was natural to give birth normally and wanted to do this.
2) I felt my recovery afterwards would be faster.

Unfortunately I ended up being induced again at 40+12 and failed to progress over 12 hours beyond 1cm. I wanted to give it some more time but found the contractions very hard to bear. I had been using my tens machine but it was not helping me to cope after 12 hours. Pethidine had given no relief and I was afraid of the Gas & Air as did not want to end up vomiting.

I wanted an epidural but they couldn't get it in after 3 attempts. I asked my Obs to do another C-section at that stage as I couldn't cope with the contractions—I was very panicky. He advised that it might be for the best in any case due to FTP and my previous c-section. So in 2004 I had my second c-section.

I have just had my third baby (by elective section) at the end of October 2009. I briefly discussed VBA2C with my Obs but he felt that it would likely end up the same way as previously. I was happy to go with another section as I recover pretty fast from them—am generally driving and moving normally after 2 weeks.

I think there is a huge reluctance to allow us to labour after caesarean and without the cooperation of our hospitals I am not sure how we can push it. Is it a fear of being sued if things go wrong that makes them stick to the 40 weeks and 12 days max over that?

I spent a lot of time researching VBAC. After the cesarean birth of my twins, at the 6 week appointment my consultant said I was a great candidate for VBAC so I just assumed I'd have one. By the time I got pregnant again I was living in a different place (Arkansas, USA), where VBAC is banned. At first I thought I'd be ok with another caesarean, but the more I thought about it, the more 'fundamentalist' I became about wanting a VBAC, and by my 12 week appointment I told my Doctor they would not cut me open. Fortunately, he is supportive, just the hospital policy is against it. So I ended up doing a lot of research, joined ICAN etc.

I am planning a VBAC for this baby for several reasons:

– Recovery time. I will have 2 year old toddler twins at home, and cannot imagine not being allowed to lift them for 6+ weeks, plus the pain in bending over to change their nappies, when having to run after them to stop them doing something etc etc.

– Future pregnancies. While it is somewhat unlikely due to age and fertility issues. We are open to the possibility of more kids. I know that the more caesareans you have, the more likely your fertility will be affected and there may be pregnancy complications.

– Statistics. Additional risk to baby in a VBAC is small. Additional risk to me in a repeat caesarean is (in my estimation) bigger. This is a big deciding factor for my husband especially.
– Emotional: While I had a good c-section experience and no regrets (it was medically necessary), I would like to experience vaginal birth, and I believe birth is not a huge medical thing and unnecessary surgery is silly.

I wanted a VBAC with my son; I'd had an emergency c section with my daughter 14 months previously. I researched risks, but in all I wanted to experience a natural birth, it never felt like I really gave birth to my daughter and I wanted the chance with my son, the hospital wouldn't allow it though, no signs of labour starting and at 41+6 I had a planned cesarean section.

Is My VBAC Just a Dream?

'Mama' is a Dublin mother of three who has chronicled her journey to 2 VBACs over three years on the popular parenting website Rollercoaster. This discussion and support for VBAC Mums still continues on Rollercoaster today.

April 4 2006:

I'm now 38 weeks pregnant and with every day it seems like my dream of a VBAC are slipping away.

All along, my hospital team have been telling me they fully support my decision for a vaginal birth, it's been 18months since my son was born by caesarean section and they didn't envisage too many complications.

So, yesterday my Doctor basically told me to forget the dream, I'm putting our lives at risk and I should just accept the fact that I'll either end up with a dangerous labour and/or a section. That either way I will need constant monitoring and some degree of intervention. Am I REALLY fooling myself? Isn't childbirth supposed to be one of the most natural things in the world? So why is it so impossible for me?

Now I just feel like running away and hiding until the baby decides to come out!

April 6th 2006

Hi girls, my head is wrecked, my due date is only a few days away and I know in my heart nothing is happening.

The Doctor basically has an answer for everything and none are the answers I want.

He knew from the start I wanted a natural birth and am willing to go more than his "10 days overdue" policy. He always said he supported my decision but now he's started trying to scare me, and belittle me actually which I'm really annoyed about

(My husband has offered to have strong words with him for upsetting me lol!)

He said he's not happy with me going more than 10 days over because I am putting my baby at risk and myself at risk. He said I can't do it naturally without some sort of intervention and wanted to know why I won't let him break my waters on my next apt (Tuesday). He said I will need to be bed restricted during labour because the baby will need constant monitoring to make sure it's not bursting out through my previous scar. He said I'm significantly increasing my risk of having a still born baby and so on and on. He's basically doing what I knew he would eventually do, trying to scare me into a section which I think is the easy way out for him, not me.

I don't know how to respond to him anymore, I haven't the strength and I'm dreading Tuesday. I know it sounds so selfish but I just wish this baby would get out cause I can't cope with the stress any more.

April 6 2006
Thanks girls - I have considered going the legal route but all this has taken me by surprise because up to now, they gave me the impression that they were all for me trying a vaginal birth, my head's spinning.

I probably sound a bit thick but I'm finding it very hard to answer him because he has an answer for everything and keeps trying to make me feel stupid or feel as though I'm being reckless with our lives. I don't have the strength to argue because it's bringing it all back to me what happened last time and my emotions are seriously getting in the way. I literally can't speak without crying now.

I've stressed to him that I'm not willing to risk our lives or our health but he says I already have a 1 in 100 chance of the baby coming out thru my old scar if I go into labour naturally and that going overdue will only increase that risk. See, I thought giving me gels, breaking my waters etc would increase this risk but he says,

"well you want me to give you a trial labour don't you?"

I said yes, but only if it happens naturally, if not I'd rather discuss a planned section without going thru anything like what I went thru last time first. So he started getting smart arsed about it saying "so now you're telling me you want a section?"

We were going round in circles basically. He said I should feel free to get a 2nd opinion but hospital policy bla bla bla...I really do feel I'd be wasting my time.

Obviously I value a Dr's medical opinion BUT I'm not convinced I've heard a valid argument against me going more than 10 days over. I don't think scare stories are helpful and I don't think him stressing me out is helpful.

I already considered "forgetting" my appointment but my husband wants to go to have words with him.

I'm just going to have to hope against hope that I miraculously go into labour before Tuesday and never have to see that Doctor again! What else can I do?

April 6
Hi ladies, thanks for all your posts.

Tuesday is his clinic day so I'll be "officially" 2 days overdue. I went 27 days over last time (which was 17 days "officially"). I thought this would work in my favour so I put it to him, look how healthy my baby was last time and he was so overdue, to which he replied: then you had more than a fair chance last time, didn't you?

I really feel there's no arguing with him and I'm not joking when I say I'm a total wreck so I'm not a good spokesperson for myself!

My husband is more than willing to speak on my behalf but is way softer than me and the Doctor will find him very easy to convince that I'm endangering me and baby. I've no doubt he'll cave, so I'll have to cave too. It's his baby & his wife and I can't argue with that?

I'd like to let him know that he's pressurising me and frankly stressing me but the last thing I want is to labelled a 'difficult patient'. I think that's a loosing battle, I'll have to think on it between now and Tuesday.

I guess what seems like a simple plan in my head baffles medical science. I tried to say to him, well, are all women on this planet designed to make a baby in exactly 40 weeks? Because I don't think I am. He pretty much laughed at me. God, do you ever wish it was still the Stone Age and medical science wasn't so "advanced" and in your face?

April 7
Hi Ladies, firstly thank you all so much for taking the time to post. I really appreciate all your opinions, whether pro VBAC or not.

Firstly, Sara, you are brave! At least you knew you'd be in for a slating! It's easy for you to be taken out of context because most of the ladies probably don't know we chat pretty much on a daily basis. I completely understand where you're coming from and thanks for that, you've been nothing but supportive to me. Yes, I do think building myself up for a v-birth has been a problem to factor in here and I totally agree with you, if it is to be a section, I'd rather it be a calmly planned one than a last minute decision that I'm not prepared for like last time. I know it would be easier to recover from mentally. That's why I'd rather avoid induction where possible. As I've said before, my last section was 18 months ago and I still haven't mentally healed.

AntiH, you haven't frightened me at all. We've chatted about our experiences in the past and I've found you to be one of the few people who actually understand what a traumatic effect a difficult birth can have on you. It's something that can be taken way too lightly. Now, I know having a section isn't the worst thing in the world and having a v-birth isn't the be all and end all of womanliness but I know you'll understand where I'm coming from when I say that a fairly 'normal' birth this time would help me psychologically more than anything? And feeling that I have some degree of control over how things pan out is also very important. At the end of the day, it's hard to explain but it's not a question of section Vs vaginal birth. I hope I'm not rambling now!

My husband & myself will attend on Tuesday of course, I'm not seriously planning on running away lol! (only in my head) I have my baby's best interests at heart first and foremost. I just have to get a bit stronger so I can stand up for myself because yes, I think the Doctor is using some degree of bully tactics. On the other hand, I totally understand he has a job to do, he wants a healthy mother and baby at the end of his shift and that he also has to comply with hospital policy, I'm fine with that. However, scaring me isn't helpful; I'd much rather that he rationally explain to me what medical procedures are needed and why. Asking me over the phone why I won't let him break my waters on Tuesday without having even examined me doesn't exactly fill me with faith.

Surely if myself and babs are fine, I'm not being irrational wanting to wait a few days more???

Thanks again ladies for all your thoughts & posts. I will of course let you know how I get on this Tuesday.

April 9
Hi Ladies, thanks again. Hubby and I have geared ourselves up for a challenge on Tuesday when we meet with the Doctor so I am currently surfing on a fact finding mission. I want to be

armed with as much information as possible. Zoof, good idea to ask him to write things down. We were discussing bringing a dictaphone.

Anyway, I'm off to do more research!

April 10
Afternoon ladies, thanks again for all your support and ideas. I googled myself half blind yesterday, so should be well prepared for tomorrow. All I need to be able to do is keep my composure.

Evie, there are a lot of valid reasons for CS and I know I will have one without a second thought if it's necessary. The most important thing to both mothers and Drs at the end of the day is a healthy baby & mammy. (If only in the physical sense) But, I have to say after what I've been thru and listening to other mothers, it seems that for every genuine case, there is a not so genuine case. WHY???

One of the books I read recently was by an ex Obs (he left the field, among other reasons, because he believes it not a place for men and is now into supporting home birthing in the UK) Anyway, at his hospital, he had gotten the CS rate down to below 7% in the 80's when CS were even more popular than they are now. He believes that most of the problems today are because pregnancy is treated as an illness and Drs aren't trained to deal with "unusual" pregnancies, that CS is the general rule.

I don't mean to ramble again but can I just say, there's a lot more to a section than the surgery itself. Once you've had one, your life and your future and the future of your family is completely changed forever and there is no going back. As I've said before, I was left very mentally scared after my 1st child, so much so that when I found out I was pregnant again I had a bit of a breakdown. Myself & my husband always said we wanted lots of children but I'm still having a hard time accepting this pregnancy and the fact that things aren't going too well isn't helping matters. I'm now faced with having to have more surgery, yes, but me & my husband may also have to come to terms with the fact that we will never be able to have another child. That's not something I ever thought I'd have to face and I feel cheated. It doesn't help that I blame myself for maybe not asking the right questions or taking more responsibility last time round. That's why it's so important to me that I do the best I can this time. This is our future we're dealing with.

April 11
God ladies, I really think my Doctor should consider changing his name to Dr Jekyll! The man I saw today was the reasonable and supportive man that I was happy to have as my Doctor in the beginning, not the man I spoke to last week!

Did the mere presence of my husband make THAT much of a difference???

So, my husband & I decided to go with our knowledge but to let him do all the talking and play along unless we disagreed with what he was saying or he got heavy with the scare tactics again.

He went through my birth plan again (which he had made notes on and signed) and explained all the parts he disagreed with and why. Lo & behold, I'm not a liar, it turns out that yes, I can get out of the bed if I'm being monitored, as I did last time! So I'm really happy we didn't have to argue about that LOL! He also said yes, he agrees with me on not wanting to have gel. I didn't have to quote the research I'd heard, he quoted it to me which was a relief. He said it's an area of great interest to him and one which he has heavily researched himself. He is aware that studies have suggested that prostaglandins can increase the risk of rupture for women with a previous caesarean and explained his opinions on the subject. He said that given my history (4 gels last time, none of which worked) that he probably wouldn't recommend it in my case this time.

Not once did he mention still born babies or my 1/100 chance of rupturing. He examined me, said that my cervix is still very unfavourable and that we would meet again to discuss my options next Tuesday (when I'll be 9 days overdue) but that if I'm still so unfavourable that I should start to prepare myself for the possibility of a section.

He stressed the importance of me & baby's wellbeing and the fact that he is very for VBACs and that he really wants me to have one.

So, all in all, we were satisfied with the meeting and I guess we just have to keep our fingers crossed for a miracle and hope that baby decides to come on its own soon...

Now, how's that for weird but wonderful!?

APMum, meant to say I'm going public. I have the option to go private but was wary of the fact that if I did, I'd be speaking to an Obs at every visit and that's not the kind of care I wanted. Last time I went public & alternated between GP and Midwife clinic which is what I prefer. Saw my Ob on my 1st visit last time and never again.

I'm totally aware that I'm at a high risk of having a section, not just because of my previous one but because I've known in my heart all along that I would go overdue with this one also, I don't know why I knew that, but I did. I knew that I'm likely to be faced with the decision to have to have a section but that's exactly what I wanted it to be my decision. Not a last minute thing after another failed induction. I have no doubt that a planned section would be much easier for me to handle physically and emotionally but I still hope that it doesn't come to that.

Anyway, here goes another week of hoping & praying

COME ON BABY!!!

April 11
Thanks again all!

I don't know why the sudden shift in persona but I'll give him the benefit of the doubt and assume he was having a really bad day last week! (???)

Anyway, I'm gonna try to get on with life a bit, enjoy my last few days with my son, give him lots of attention, he deserves it. Poor boy has had a blubbering mad woman for a mama lately LOL!

I'm not giving up on the old wives tales yet. I'll still be drinking my raspberry leaf tea, bouncing on inflatable furniture (and hubby if I'm lucky) because you just never know, this could be my week!

Anyway, hopefully I'll be posting a positive birth story soon, whatever the final outcome.

Thanks ladies!
M

April 18
Well, had my appointment this morning and I'm afraid it's not looking good. Basically, I am still "unfavourable" and due to my history and the risks involved with induction (namely, the use of prostaglandins), he wants me to come in on Friday morning for a section.

Time and hope is rapidly running out and I'm really fighting a losing battle at this stage. He can't offer me any explanation as to why I'm not yet ready to give birth and to be honest, I find that the most frustrating thing of all. Surely my theory, that maybe I take longer than 40 weeks to make a baby and we should let nature take its course is a better one than "it happens to some women"???

I'm devastated to say the least; we're not sure where to go from here.

April 18
Thanks ladies. I don't see the point in mentioning it to my Doctor but I do want to get a 2nd opinion. I obviously want to make sure 1st & foremost that my baby is born safe & well. As of today, plenty of movement, good strong heartbeat, plenty of fluid etc... But I can't shake the niggling feeling that there's something not right about being told that some women just fail to give birth...

April 23
Ladies, I have to say, I never thought I would be sitting here writing this. Just a quick note to say, my waters broke in the early hours of Thursday morning. We went to the hospital soon after when my contractions were 4mins apart. Against all the odds, I gave birth to my beautiful little daughter at 3:42 that afternoon!

I am so happy that I can't even put it into words! It was so amazing! This time, every time I relive the birth I can't stop crying tears of JOY!

Now, I have a lovely baby to admire...will log on again asap.

Just wanted to say thanks again for all the encouragement you all gave me.

M

▍ Mama's 2ⁿᵈ VBAC

April 2008—I can't believe it was more than 2 years ago that I posted this thread!

My little princess was 2 years old yesterday. Again, it made me think of all these emotions.

Thanks again to all of you who helped me through it!
And good luck to all of you who are waiting on your VBAC!

Caoilagh's Birth

Monday 1st—The braxton hicks I'd been having started to change. They were much stronger and were now accompanied with lower back pain. In the evening, they got stronger and more frequent. I went to bed but couldn't sleep with the pain in my back. Zac was doing all the right things, offering me a back rub, he got me my ball to sit on but it made my back pain worse, he asked me if I wanted to listen to my CD and I said no, it would annoy me. He asked me if I wanted a bath and I said no, I was too uncomfortable. Getting into the early hours the surges were very irregular but very strong and the pressure was unreal! By 3am the pain in my back was too bad, I thought we would have to go to the hospital. Zac called my sister in Dublin and she arrived out in a Taxi around 4:30am. She went to bed and I told her I'd let her know when we were leaving. After that, things seemed to slow down. Zac went back to bed, the time between surges paced out and I was nodding off in between.

Tuesday 2nd—By morning I only had back pain and small surges every 20 / 30 minutes. The kids went to their childminder and Zac went to work. Not much happened the rest of the day so I went to bed to catch up on my sleep. By Tuesday evening things started to ramp up again.

Again the surges got stronger and more frequent, the pressure was still there and the pain in my back was getting really bad. I knew that being difficult the previous night hadn't helped so I told Zac to keep doing what he was doing and encouraging me to focus on relaxing. I listened to my CD and had a bath. I found a comfortable chair to sit in and watched some comedy on TV. We went to bed early in case anything happened and my sister stayed over again. Again the surges got really strong and I sat in bed watching, amazed at how the force of them lifted my whole bump off my lap! The pain in my back got more intense. Zac put my CD on repeat, he ran me a bath and we lit some candles. After a while Zac went to bed and I stayed in the bath for about 4 hours, it felt great. Eventually, things died down again and I went to bed around 6am.

Wednesday 3rd—The kids went to their childminder again. I had an antenatal appointment at the Midwives clinic at 12 and Zac came with me. When I went to collect my urine sample I had a show. I was delighted something new was happening! I was lost mid-surge when the Midwife called me to come in. She asked was I having pains and joked that I was in the wrong place if I was in labour. The Midwife reminded me that I should go to hospital sooner rather than later as I needed IV antibiotics for StrepB infection. We went home feeling a little more optimistic that things might actually be happening. Wednesday seemed to be panning out the same as the nights before and I was very downhearted. The pain in my back was bad; baths didn't offer as much relief. The surges were unbelievably strong and yet not painful. I listened to my Gentlebirth CD on repeat, surfed the net, read a book, but couldn't sleep.

Thursday 4th—Around 6am I suddenly got a burst of energy. I got up, got washed and dressed, even put on some make-up. I woke Zac and told him I wanted to go to hospital. He got up and got ready while I packed the last few bits and pieces in my bag.

I told my sister we were going and off we went. I knew Zac was annoyed that I was going to make him miss another days work. I put on my CD in the car and slept most of the way to the hospital getting surges every 8—10 minutes. We arrived at the hospital at 8am, the sight of the place made me queasy. Zac asked if I wanted to wait a while in the car but I was feeling confident. We went in and booked into admissions. They asked me was I having pains and I said yes, although, apart from the constant pain in my back, I wasn't having 'pains' just tightenings.

We were brought to the labour ward; to the same bed I had the last time which made me feel a little uneasy. The Midwife came and introduced herself and spent ages going through my birth plan with us. She told me that because I was having a VBAC, they'd prefer me to be on a constant trace throughout labour and that the hospital had a rule to check dilation every 2 hours but that didn't have to be strictly enforced depending on how we were doing. There was no problem with anything else in the birth plan. She asked what classes we had done and I told her gentlebirth. She said she had seen hypno births and "it really does work". I found that reassuring!

So, she put me on the routine admissions trace and said if it was ok she would be back in 20/30 mins and "check to see if anything's happening". While we waited I told Zac that once I knew everything was ok he could drop me home and go on to work as it was still early. I knew he dreaded hours or days of waiting around the hospital again so that perked him up.

The Midwife came back and checked the trace, baby was fine, small contractions about every 10mins. I said it was ok to check me and she did. I was 5cms! Not the news we expected at all! The Midwife said "see, the hypnobirthing does work!" The consultant Professor came in and introduced herself and confirmed everything the Midwife had said and wished me luck.

So, I was moved to the delivery room, the same room where I had my daughter last year. Myself and Zac both stopped at the door and looked at each other; it didn't bring back good memories. Zac asked the Midwife if there was a different room and she said they were all the same. We reluctantly went in. I perched myself on the side of the bed and put on my headphones. My Midwife came in and introduced herself, she was soon joined by another who introduced herself. They'd had a look at my file and birth plan. The second Midwife quickly establishing herself as a real character said to me "I don't care if you want to give birth standing on your head. We're not here to tell you what to do, we're only here to help you if you need us. You listen to your body and do what it tells you." So far so good I thought! I told her I remembered her from when I had my daughter last year. She asked was that good or bad and I said definitely good.

Her face is the one thing I always remembered about the birth of my daughter. In the sea of people telling me I wasn't progressing, I needed a section, nothing was happening etc etc, she kept popping her head in and saying "you can do this Louise, I know you can".

The Midwife asked me did I want to put on a nightdress or pyjamas and I said no. She put me on the trace and the antibiotic drip was set up. As I sat and listened to my CD and relaxed the space between surges started to increase, I decided to ignore the time and concentrate on my relaxation. I told Zac he should go for some air or a coffee before things started happening. He left and I sat on the bed and nodded off as the Midwives came in and out of the room. Things were ticking along nicely and my confidence was building.

Around 12:15 one Midwife asked me how I was feeling. I said I felt fine except for the pain in my back. She asked if I'd like her to check my dilation, I hadn't been checked since 9am. I said no and she said that was no problem, she didn't want to be doing internals or breaking waters if I didn't want it. She said that's no problem, she had no reason to be checking me if I didn't want it. She suggested I straddle a chair to see if it eased the pain in my back and said the position would help to open the pelvis and help the baby down and that it might even encourage my waters to break. She got me a chair and put a pillow over the back of it. I rested my head and continued listening to my CD. The pain in my back quickly got worse and another Midwife started to rub it for me, Zac came back and took over the back rub. The pain soon got too bad so I had to stand up. I perched on the edge of the bed and Zac went round the other side to rub my back. The Midwife bent to fix the trace back in place and I felt like an elastic band snapped in my belly. I said "oh, I think my waters are going" I felt another elastic band snap, heard a pop and my waters released in a sudden warm gush! I couldn't believe the amount of liquid! I was soaked, the Midwife, bent in front of me was soaked, and there was a huge puddle on the floor. I started apologising for the mess, the Midwife was busy cleaning and reassuring me.

I said "wow, did you hear that pop when they released!?" but I was the only one that heard it. I felt silly for being so over-whelmed and I said to the Midwife how I thought it was amazing but I suppose she must see that happen every day. But she said no, that was the first time she'd seen a woman's waters release spontaneously, and that most women here have their waters broken for them.

The surges suddenly started to come very quickly, 4 or 5 in a row with only a minute or so between. They felt different, more intense, and biggeA few minutes later, the Midwife came back and asked if I wanted to get up on the bed, that I could kneel and lean over the back of it so I did. She was delighted that my waters had released on their own and said that it probably wouldn't be long and that my contractions would be much more frequent now.

The surges continued, strong and frequent and there was im-
mense pressure at the peak of each one. The pressure was overwhelming and I could hear myself making a strange grunting
noise with each one! The 3rd Midwife came in, and asked me
if I felt like pushing, I said no, I feel pressure. She said "can I
check you, we can't have you pushing down on a cervix that
isn't fully open or you will do yourself a serious injury". She
said "will you lie down and let me check you?" The pressure
was so intense I wondered if it was the baby's head and got worried that things were happening too fast. I asked her if I needed
to lie down or if she could check me in the position I was in. She
said she could check me where I was. Before I knew what was
happening she had given me the roughest, most painful internal
and I screamed in pain. I heard her snap off her gloves and say
to the other Midwife, "she's only 6cms there's nothing happening there" and she left the room. I turned to Zac, "did she say
I'm only 6cms?" He nodded. I felt sure I had dilated more. A
few minutes later, a Doctor appeared at the bed. He said your
Midwife told me you haven't progressed since 9am so what we
would like to do is get you started on a drip and we would like
to take a sample of blood from the baby's scalp to see how it is
doing. I looked at Zac as I breathed thru another surge. It was
obvious he couldn't believe what he was hearing either! He said
"NO! We don't want any of that, I'll ask Louise but I'm certain
she won't want any of that" I told the Doctor I didn't want any
of that; he just stood there looking at me. I said to Zac I have
dilated 6cms, my waters have gone on their own, I'm getting
strong, regular contractions, how dare he say I'm not making
progress. The Doctor left the room. I told the Midwife I needed
the bathroom.

Zac and I went into the bathroom and he held me. There was no
need for the brutality that woman had just shown me. I couldn't
stop crying. I felt violated and assaulted and degraded and de-
moralised. I couldn't understand why they were suddenly telling
me I wasn't making progress when to me, I obviously was.

Zac said I needed to ignore it and get my focus back. I was making progress. I told him I would go back out, get back on the bed and he could put my headphones on from behind and rub my back. We went back out. I stood by the bed and sucked on the Gas & Air as I had another strong surge. The 3rd Midwife arrived back in the room; she asked me again if I felt like pushing, I said no. She said I want you to get back on the bed; you can't have your baby standing there. She was instructing the other Midwife to get things prepared for the baby. I was trying to focus and she was going on and on "if you push standing there, your baby will fall onto the hard floor, it has happened. Women can go from 6 to 10 centimetres very quickly.

I need you to get back onto the bed." She came towards me and started to try to push me up onto the bed. The other Midwife stepped in and told her to let me get up myself, which I did. The not so nice Midwife led her out of the room and I told Zac to please not let her come back in near me.

Zac put my headphones back on and I tried to concentrate but they fell off as I had a surge. I wanted Zac to put pressure on my back rather than try to get the headphones on. The surges were so intense and now I could feel my body pushing down. I started to fight against it. The Midwife came in and asked me did I need to push and I said yes but I was trying not to. She said no, do whatever my body was telling me to do. I said "but the other Midwife just told me not to push because I was only 6cms and I'd do myself an injury". She tried to reassure me to listen to my body. She said if my body was telling me to push that I should push.

I told her I was afraid of doing myself an injury. She said I should trust my body and that she had been a Midwife 25 years and I could trust her. She said if it made me feel better she would check me again to see if I was fully dilated. I couldn't face another internal. I was too upset and confused now and my body was doing its own thing and pushing down with each surge.

I couldn't stop it, I'd lost control. I can't describe how intense the surges were at this stage. They were so powerful they physically moved my whole body forcing me back into a squat.

I quickly got tired and told Zac to ask for the epidural. The Midwife said she would have to check me to see if there was time and I agreed. I didn't feel her check me but she did and told me she could feel the baby's head, there was no time for an epidural. Each surge came more powerfully than the last and I was exhausted and feeling sick. It was time to push. I turned around onto my back and continued to push with the surges. I looked at the Midwife; she was sweating and looked worried. She said the baby was stuck and was passing meconium. She told called a Paediatrician to come and continued encouraging me to push. She said that the baby would get tired soon and I had to keep trying. She was worried about my previous tear, the scar looked very weak and she was concerned that if I tore it again it would be very bad. They hurried around getting things ready and encouraging me to push down with each surge. "Your baby is showing signs of distress and passing meconium and I have 2 consultants outside the door that want to forceps your baby out. I don't want that to happen so you have to push for me. Forget about the Gas and just concentrate on your breathing and pushing, I know you can do this, you're doing great."

Zac took the gas and I tried to focus, to visualise my baby moving closer with each surge, to imagine it slipping out easily. I could hear the baby's heart rate regular and strong on the monitor, at one point Susie said she'd never seen a child so happy being born, the heart rate was great, it was almost like it was enjoying being born! I continued pushing with each surge and was feeling queasy and tired. I remember one Midwife saying to the other "that was transition, that was the strangest transition I've ever seen" I wish I had asked her later what she meant by that!

The Midwife said she could see the baby's head coming closer each time I pushed. She asked did we bring a mirror to see it. No, NOT the type of thing I would want to see! She said baby had a lovely head of hair and I should touch the head which I did.

She said baby would be here in a few minutes but again she was very worried about my scar, it was really under pressure and she asked me what I wanted to do. I knew I didn't want it to tear again so I told her to go ahead with an episiotomy if it looked as though it was going to give. She said if she really had to, she would do a very small snip. I tried to get in a better position and continued to follow through as my body pushed. She kept on encouraging me as one of the consultants (professor) arrived and she explained what was happening. "It's not a small baby she's having." The consultant nodded and smiled at me but otherwise just stood by and let Susie work. I felt a stinging sensation, then I felt the snip of the episiotomy and the head was out. The Midwife asked if I wanted her to tell me the sex of the baby, I said no. One more push and the rest of the baby was born. She handed me my baby, white from head to toe, a little girl. "I shouldn't really do this with the Paediatrician waiting but I know you want the cord to stop pulsating. I held my baby and when the cord stopped pulsating she went to hand "Daddy" the scissors. I thought he would pass out! I said I would cut her cord. They took baby away to be checked over by the Paed, she was fine.

Ironically, the Midwife later came in and hugged me and apologised to me for "being such a bitch". She said she just didn't want me to have any interventions, she knew I could do it without any. She literally had to hold back the Doctors from coming in with their forceps and I thanked her for that. She was far from a bitch, I thought she was fantastic. I only wish all Midwives were like her.

I know it's not the most successful Gentlebirth story but I really feel it did help me. Without it, I don't think I would have laboured at home for so long.

If it's any comfort, apart from the back pain, I was never in any real pain with the surges, the best way I can describe them is "intense". I believe that had I been in a better position, my body would have pushed my baby out itself without any help from me, that's how intense it was. Even towards the end when I had no pain relief, the Episiotomy didn't hurt. As my daughter was being born I felt a strong stinging sensation, not something I would describe as painful though, very much the opposite of my last experience when I was screaming in agony for the epidural at 2cms!

If it hadn't been for that one 'bad apple', if I hadn't let what she did shake my confidence and the sense of control my birth experience may have turned out very differently.

Caoilagh was born at 3.22pm last Thursday

▌ Rotunda VBAC

I can't believe it's taken me two weeks to sit and share this story but things are definitely busier with three boys!

Two weeks ago today Conor Francis arrived after a natural labour using hypnobirthing and an amazing doula!

First a little history... Five years ago we welcomed our first son into the world using hypnobirthing. It was a long (22 hours) but gentle labour, most of which I spent at home. Labouring naturally, without drugs and listening to my body was an incredible experience and one I definitely wanted to repeat. So discovering I had complete placenta previa on my second pregnancy and had no choice but to have a c-section was very disappointing for me. But this is just the beginning of the story!

Pregnant for a third time (now with no complications) I first found that amazing Irish doula who helped me find a very VBAC friendly consultant. Our discussion of the birth plan went well and he seemed totally on board with all my 'no intervention' requests.

Saturday afternoon (two days after my due date) my waters began to leak and I got excited that I was finally going to meet our third boy! I texted Tracy who assured me that labour probably wouldn't get started until I had put our other boys to bed! She was so right... by 8pm the house was quiet. I took out my CD, sat on my ball, dimmed the lights and began to relax. By 10 pm I knew I was in active labour and felt ready for Tracy's company. I laboured at home, peacefully until 2am when a particularly strong surge told me it was time to head to the Rotunda.

My heart sank when, after a Midwife checked me, I was 'only' 3cm. But once I was in the delivery room upstairs Tracy helped me focus quickly and I soon forgot the tone of the Midwife downstairs. I shut out everything around me and focused on Tracy's voice (way better than any CD!) and two hours later (seemed like 20 minutes) I was 9cm! My surges were very strong at the end and never closer than 6 minutes apart but I found that visualizing the baby's journey down really helped. At 6.40am I gave birth to a beautiful, healthy 8lb little boy.

So although this labour and birth was very different to my first, hypnobirthing was again a vital tool in bringing Conor naturally and peacefully into the world.

Oh and one more thing... Just as I would never climb Mount Everest without a sherpa, I would never have another natural birth without a doula!

▌ VBAC

I had my first false start 6 days pre-due date, in over night and home again, second false start 4 days pre-due date. I was seen at 40 weeks and was told we would discuss induction or section at next app. I decided to try some acupuncture and booked it for sat afternoon. Was getting plenty of pains but nothing that was sticking. On Sat more pains and longer and stronger so I call my mil to come down as the weather was too bad for her to travel at night. The acupuncturist came at 2pm did her stuff and I was still getting short pains about 20—25 min apart. I had a show at 6:30 and pains increased to 15 mins apart. I watched X-factor and headed into the hospital.

It was so disappointing to be only 2-3cms and not in labour. After a consensual sweep, my husband went to my Mother in Laws and I settled into the ward at midnight. I put on my CD and relaxed totally for an hr and a half by 2:30 I was getting 1 min pains 5 minutes apart and increasing in frequency, was still working through but as I was only 3cms I decided I wanted some pain relief. Off to the delivery suite I woke up my husband and he arrived. By 3am I was in labour, pains coming fast and strong, between each one I struggled to relax at first but then I settled into a rhythm and could bring myself almost to the point of sleep for a few seconds.

I took some gas and air and as I was still not even 4cms I asked for and epidural. They had to break waters for that and the pain got very intense, but further apart. When the Doctor came at 4:35 to do the epidural, I was starting to push; I was fully dilated and ready to go. Between each contraction I was able to completely relax and repeated the affirmations in my head to bolster my confidence. gas and air abandoned, I started to push actively at near 5am. After each push I dived mentally into my relaxation place and prepared for the next one. One at a time, I could do anything for 1 minute and I could do anything for an hour was all I could say in my head.

My little girl arrived into the world at 6:30 on the button, facing the wrong way to everyone's surprise. I had a small tear, but I had the almost completely natural birth I dreamed off. Great Midwives and fantastic husband were really important parts of the experience.

▌ Our First VBAC—Dublin

I was kept in Unit 3 on Wednesday night (26th March) due to pre-eclampsia worries. It was very busy and as I had been drinking so much water (trying to get a negative protein sample!) I was up every hour to pee- plus there was already "pressure" on my bladder. I had to share a cubicle with another patient, that's how busy it was...

I asked to go home on Thursday as I was exhausted and the sounds of other ladies going into labour all night was definitely not the sort of "Zen" pre-birth experience I had been hoping for....

I slept so well on Thursday night. I had to go back to day ward on Friday and unfortunately still lots of protein in urine and BP raised (not too high, but enough). I was kept in again. Hadn't thought it would happen so had nothing with me!!

I was devastated. I just sat on the bed in Unit 3 and cried. Then I realised there was lots I could still do and to get a grip. I was terrified though. Got my husband to come in with bags, and he brought an acupuncturist. I got it done even though it terrifies me. Started sniffing clary sage and had a huge pineapple on my bedside locker..... Started having pains that night, they were about every 30 mins, severe painful bladder pressure (not in "cervix" as such) making me feel like I had to run to loo constantly, even if I didn't need to go. They would come in waves, three together and then nothing for 30 mins. Didn't sleep too well that night.

Saturday: Kids came in to see me; bored senseless- wanting sweets and running about. Having on and off really horrid bladder pressure all day long. Couldn't rest with it as I couldn't lie down, too painful to get up. That night, I got moved to a quieter room- the Midwives were fab, giving me that room! Only problem was now *I* was the one making the noise. Bladder pressure pains very sore. That night they turned into more frequent contraction type pains for about 2 hours before tapering off. Baby was jumping about all this time in between like crazy-0 really violent swishes and even what felt like savage "head butts" on my groin/bladder.

About 1am I was not coping well and the pains—still well and truly doing nothing, I just knew, were so intense and I was SO tired I just was crying out loud in the loo. They were very intense and then would dissipate totally for about half an hour. So frustrating as well. The Midwife heard me and asked to do a VE. I agreed and she said I was "in labour" I asked if I was dilated and if not to leave me as I really wanted to wait on account of not being given to long in labour ward with my VBAC. She said I was "well on" but wouldn't say how far.

I texted my husband and went to the labour ward. Walked though the doors and the pains disappeared—stopped cold! The Midwife asked was I having any pains and I said no. Did a CTG trace for an hour and I slept so soundly- best 9and only sleep I'd had in 2 days. I explained the VBAC thing again and asked if I was dilated. She said I was very favourable but no. THANKS BE TO GOD!!

Sunday: pottered about like a fool, rather than rest because... at 5pm, pains in bladder area again thick and fast. Felt bad making noise in quiet room, and too much to bear so stood in shower until 1am. Sat in the chair in the shower room in my soaking robe falling asleep between pains (every 5 mins, but all in bladder, not in vagina) until daybreak.

Monday: The pains were gone for most part. The Obstetrician came to see me. He did a VE (still favourable, still 2cm) I was absolutely shattered, physically, emotionally. He discussed rupturing membranes the next day. I wanted to wait longer but the thoughts of doing another night like the one before was terrifying too. I made lots of phone calls. My husband came in to see me, pains starting up again. Called a friend and asked her advice—she suggested a doula and I thought it would be a good idea. I also called a homeopath suggested by another friend and she set me at ease too- even just telling her how I felt and how I really wanted this VBAC but was terrified of the pain/ yet more pain... She suggested some remedies for clearing the blockages I had due to fear.

The doula arrived and she set me at ease straight away. She said she wouldn't leave me and it was just was I needed to hear. I had felt so alone and here was someone who would be with me. The Midwives are so busy and they were mainly limited to checking if I was ok, and doing medical stuff, and asking about the pains, which of course, I was being cagey about lest I end up in the labour ward (again) too soon. All night long, I had contractions and finally they felt like they were doing something. Sat on chair all night with doula helping me breathe and focus the energy to opening my cervix. So hard to do. Again I fell asleep between contractions and it felt like they were 30 mins apart as I was asleep, but she said they were getting closer and in the end only 2-3 mins apart and over minute long.

The Midwife came in a few times and I was telling her they were still irregular as I wasn't to wait until dawn- everything is more manageable in daylight. When she came in to do CTG monitoring at 6.30 I couldn't hide the fact the contractions were every few minutes.

Tuesday: Down to labour ward. Walked through the doors once again and the pains stopped totally! From 3 mins apart to NOTHING. I was petrified, I was exhausted, I wanted to run away. My doula said I needed to get control back and get contractions up again. I tried, but I had to clear my head space again. VE and lo and behold, after that night...2 f*cking centimetres and very favourable. Just focussed and mind over matter and slowly the contractions started coming back. The Midwife said that sometimes happens and that was reassuring that she believed it too. Then they broke my waters and contractions thick and fast. Breathing through them, very hard with construction workers outside being noisy.

But the window was open and the cool Spring air was wafting in and it was so sunny and I thought- what a day to be born!!

3 hours after waters broken (and continuous monitoring). I was on the birth ball the whole time. I detest those high beds. Had a VE again and I was still 2 cm. I took the Entonox to get up on the bed (I had tried this on last 2 labours and it hadn't worked but I hadn't been using it properly- OMG!!! That stuff should NOT be legal!) and I was high as a kite and talking sh*te! Doula (and Midwife) were laughing at my nonsense and it was lovely to break the tension! At that point though I asked for the epidural as my time was running out and I said to my doula "I tried" and I really had- 3 nights of difficult pains, no sleep, breathing and great contractions...and still only 2cm.

But then, as the anaesthetist was siting the needle I felt the urge to push. He said that happens sometimes with epidural and I was saying ok at first, and then NO this is different"!!!!! The Midwife checked me again (bear in mind this is less than an hour after last VE) and I was 6cm!! (Maybe I just needed to accept everything happening to me and finally surrender). The epidural never really took (could feel all the ice on the ice test) but it was just enough to take the edge off and I still had my gasssssssssssssssssssssss. (now I had to use it to NOT focus energy to my vagina, after all that!)

An hour later I was fully dilated! Then I was asked to push as baby still high. Gave an almighty push and sister said WAIT we have to get everything ready!!- he was going whoosh!- had to pant thru next 2 contractions and then 4 pushes and he was out. It was amazing. As I had thought I would end up with caesarean again, my husband was in with me and he was there for the birth. I felt on top of the world. I couldn't believe it. The Midwife asked "was a VBAC really so important to you?" (puzzled, like, not mean) and I said YES!!!!!!!!!!!!!! and girls it was marvellous. I am still in awe, and amazement that it happened for me.

I was able to get up nearly straight away- shower, hold my son, I felt a million quid. I went to the shop to get the day's paper and I felt like shouting out around the whole hospital.

Girls, I would advise you. Follow what you want, use everything available to you. The one affirmation I kept chanting in my mind was "you CAN do it".

▌ Our 2nd VBAC

Following is our 2nd VBAC story. In 2010 the Doctor told me I had a 60% chance of VBAC even though I'd had no problems with the last VBAC.

So, Sunday morning my son came in to our bed about 6.30 or 7.30am and I noticed I was getting my bladder pains shortly after that. I put on my Hypno thing (Mp3) and lay in bed. Then my daughter came in and she and my little boy were jumping all over the bed, and I was cross, so I got up and jumped in shower.

Bladder pains were very sore and so I decided to go to my Dad's to help out after making the brekkie for distraction. Went over and was a bit useless, as pains every 2-3 mins, but felt like only lasting maybe 15 seconds or so. Still convinced they were bladder pains like on my second son, and breathing through them.

I didn't feel like doing too well, so I texted my doula and asked her to come out (she'd already suggested getting into the bath to see what that would do). So dropped Dad to mass at 11.30 and then headed home.

My husband ran the bath, lit a few candles and I got in with 2 paracetamol, a glass of water and my MP3 player. Still felt like short little pains, and mainly bladder but then thought about it and tummy was hardening, but couldn't feel anything much "down below" if you get me, so thought not much of it.

My doula arrived just before 1. She said I was having contractions lasting 50 seconds and every 2-3 mins. Lay down into the bath then and felt reasonably manageable breathing through it. Bloody window in bathroom was broken and snow was blowing in!! No concept of time really, but after a bit I felt like things were getting on a bit and I would like to get to the hospital. Asked my doula to get my husband to get the kids collected (they were running up and down the hall yelling and slamming doors!) A few contractions (but what felt like a zillion years) later, felt a pop, then on next contraction felt waters coming out. Really wanted to go then. Feeling more and more urge to push, but really just couldn't believe it and just thought, ok, time to head in (and get my entonox). Then urge even stronger and my husband still yelling at kids to put shoes on!!! I asked for an ambulance.

Then got up on my knees and I knew he was coming out!! Out he popped, really fast, 2 contractions (one for head, one for body) and then after that the ambulance arrived. Went in to delivery ward—got my entonox!—really surreal experience to be in there already holding my baby! Delivered placenta and so on.

All went well and we're delighted.

Some afterthoughts on my unplanned Home VBAC

When I first notice the contractions, I just put them down to "pressure pains" like I had with my second son and I was simply trying to distract myself. I was breathing and leaning over cushions and stuff. When I realised that I was actually having real contractions, then I was sort of glad because I knew that I wouldn't be endlessly waiting for the "real deal" to start. I got in to the bath at this stage and it was fine with the breathing and the water.

I was listening to the GentleBirth CD (on MP3)- although I felt totally confident about VBAC anyway, plus I was way more relaxed and thought que sera sera this time- I have already had a great VBAC.

I was just generally more relaxed this time (I had such stress last time in re trying for my VBAC that I was keyed up like crazy). After a little bit I put the CD on to the music track and I found I could just drift off between contractions (something I was never really able to do before). My doula arrived about one and we just kept going. Anytime I felt I was going off track she was there to bring me back on track.

By the time I felt like I would like to get to the hospital I was probably about 20 mins away from having him- I already felt a bit of pushing pressure and then next thing my waters went, so I though I should go to the hospital then. I wasn't scared in the least, I just wanted my entonox!!! I was feeling really good— more like I was in the moment- I wasn't really feeling any way at all if that makes sense? The only reason I was a bit freaked was because the baby hadn't kicked for ages and I was a bit worried about that.

He was coming and there wasn't anything I could do just go with it, and that's what I did. I knew my Doula was there anyway and would help me through it.

Afterwards there was just a feeling of disbelief and incredulity (incredulousness?) that he was actually here, in my arms and it was all over. How great!

It was a really great experience.

▍ Our Perfect VBAC

I'm still in a state of blissed out shock, but I got my perfect VBAC on Tuesday, and sitting here with my gorgeous little girl Sophia Rose.

Had been getting Braxton hicks for a few days, and woke on Tuesday morning (was due on Monday) with really mild but very regular cramps. They were so mild, and I was in flying form, I really wasn't sure of this was it. This was 5.30am, and by 6.30 they were every 10 minutes, so I woke my husband and we rang the mothers to collect my son, and I texted my Doula, Caroline. I thought I'd be at home for hours at this stage. The cramps stayed the same intensity, but by 8.30am were every 5 minutes. Caroline arrived and we made a coffee, it was just so relaxed, and everyone was in great form. I still couldn't believe it was labour. I'd been induced with my son, and there is just no comparing the pain. I kept thinking I had called everyone in for no reason!

I rang the hospital just to let them know I'd be in later, but they said to think about coming in now, as it may happen fast being my second labour. So we drove in, and arrived. But as soon as I got in the contractions slowed down. I was disappointed to find that I'd have to be monitored throughout the labour, being a previous CS. I'd hoped to be able to walk about outside and take showers etc. I was 3cm, but things had kind of tailed off, and the Doctors were talking oxytocin drips etc. NO WAY! (I felt that was the quickest way to another section and wanted to avoid any intervention).

So me and Caroline took the task in hand, and I started squatting, she started acupressure and the contractions kicked off again. I zoomed through dilation, the pain was still so bearable (and I'm a WUSS with pain), I was amazed. I was enjoying every second of it! It felt so natural, unlike the induction which felt terrifyingly out of my control and overwhelming.

At about 7cm my waters broke, and the pains started getting stronger. Tried a puff of gas and air, but waste of time—I had to sit down with it, which I hated, so wheeled that away. Caroline was pressing points on my back which really helped, because those big contractions felt almost too much. The baby was still very high up though and was facing sideways, and by 9cm the baby was still so high they mentioned the 'c' word again, and I was so deflated. The pains had gotten suddenly so intense, and I was roaring like a lion throughout, felt like I was exploding!

I couldn't believe I'd gotten so far, only to have it snatched away at the last second. I also reckoned because my contractions were so strong and I was hopping all over the place with them, that a spinal block would be out of the question and I'd probably need a general—I was crest fallen—my lifetime dreams of a magical vaginal birth were about to be taken away from me forever.

So the Midwife said she's see how I'd get on for the next short while and make a decision. She left the room, and I decided I weren't accepting that! I started squatting again, and really focusing on getting the baby in the right position, even giving a sneaky push to ease her down, and Caroline used some special acupressure points. I actually felt the baby move into place, but daren't hope just in case. The Midwife came back, back up on the bed and she checked me—baby was down and facing the right way!!! She told me to start pushing, but I still didn't know if this was it, and that I'd avoided a section. So I started pushing (what a relief—pushing took over that massive pain). I have to say at this point girls, this was the reason me and my husband decided he wouldn't be there—I just couldn't have let go enough with him there—you really have to leave your dignity at he door and throw everything at that pushing!! After what felt like an hour, the Midwife said to feel down, and I touched the top of her little head. At this point I asked if I was going to do it, no section? She said yes, and I was so thrilled! Pushed some more, and looked down to see my amazing little daughter come out and straight on my chest! Girls, my heart EXPLODED!

My husband came in to the lovely calm aftermath, and sat with our little girl while I was stitched up (ow—deffo worst bit haha!). What bliss! Sophia Rose was 8lb 2oz, and labour lasted about 8 hours, only about 2 of which were tough. What a difference natural labour was to the induction!

This whole experience has put all the ghosts of my son's birth to rest. I'm an oddball in that I've looked forward to labour and giving birth since I was little!! The Midwives were brilliant, and helped me through every step (even fending off the Doctor and trigger happy oxytocin use)! And my Doula Caroline was just brilliant—she pulled me through and kept me going—not sure I'd have been able to keep going without her support. And it meant my husband actually enjoyed the experience too, knowing she was minding me. Even the Midwives, who were highly suspicious of her when she arrived, were looking to employ her at the end!!

Whilst I'm in no hurry to repeat the experience, and think I must have left my pelvic floor somewhere—can't find it anywhere... it truly was the most empowering, rewarding and life affirming experiences of my life and I'll cherish it forever!

Good luck to those trying for VBACs—reading other people's success stories helped me so much. You can do it too!

▌ Daniel's Birth Story - Wonderful VBAC

On the 22nd March I visited an acupuncturist in the hope of avoiding a chemical induction in hospital and so reducing my chances of a VBAC. It was a relaxing session and I enjoyed it immensely despite being nervous to start with. The next day I had a check up and was told though changes were afoot, I would not go into labour today or tomorrow. The doctor, however agreed with my decision not to be induced until at least 14 days over so I was delighted with that and agreed I'd come back to the hospital at 9 days over for a scan and to check both my self and baby were doing well. I relaxed and myself and my husband went to a pub for some grub and I had a glass of wine, before picking up my DD from crèche. It was a lovely sunny day and we enjoyed eating outside.

Interestingly, in my mind movie I had prepared for birth, I had said it was a lovely day and we ate outside before I had contractions!
Anyway, that night we went to bed and My husband gave me some of his own prostaglandin and headed off for a long sleep. I woke at 4am however to the feeling of the first surge. Out comes the mobile to time them, ten mins later – another one, ten mins later another….

I got excited and told My husband who was somewhat disbelieving and put his hand on my tummy. By the time the next one came he was asleep again! By 5.30 I was too excited to sleep so I got up and watched TV and went on the internet to share my expectations with fellow April Mammies.

This continued through the morning and next day and My husband went off to work. I spent the day with My sister and we went for a short walk, played with my DD and I took some short naps listening to my gentlebirth tracks. After My husband came home we called My brother to stay the night and he arrived at 8.30. At this stage I was still getting surges at 10 mins apart but they seemed stronger. By 10.30 I was getting worried about the baby and why I was having surges for so long but nothing was changing.

We agreed to go to the Rotunda to get checked out but if I was less than 3 cm to return home. We packed the car and headed off, stopping once to get over a strong surge.

Thankfully the hospital was a mere 15 minutes drive away so we timed the departure for just after a contraction! When we got to the Rotunda, we were sent into the emergency room and eventually checked.
I was 4 cms and told I was in labour and would be brought to the delivery ward.. Great! I was hooked up to a trace for 20 minutes which I found irritating as it is so much harder to deal with a surge lying down.

After a while a midwife came into me and asked me if I had discussed my birthplan with a registrar in the ante natal clinic and I said I had. She said it had a few things in it that would be outside of hospital protocol and she was surprised this hadn't been raised with me. (it had but I wasn't going to change my plan! And I had been given varied responses from each professional I had spoken to about it in the clinic anyway!) So a doctor was sent for who eventually came down and highlighted the key problem areas as refusing continuous monitoring and the time limits placed on labour. We discussed why I didn't want continuous monitoring as I didn't want m movements restricted in labour and wanted to use a shower if needed but the time limits discussion was the most fraught. She was unhappy with my calling time limits arbitrary and informed me in a not too friendly manner that they deliver x number of babies a year and their research shows that long labour leads to increased maternal and infant morbidity and mortality.

She asked me if I was willing to be in labour for 24 hours or for my child to be flat lining at birth or to have cerebral palsy? What a thing to say! Of course, I had to say, yes I am. I explained that I am not irresponsible but will not have my labour timed as long as both myself and baby were doing well and there was no indicator of distress. Anyway, eventually she covered her self with detailed patient notes which outlined what I had been informed of and my decision and we both signed it.

So off to the delivery suite, room 1, where the midwives also said that they would prefer for me to be continuously monitored but that they would agree to monitor me every 14 mins or so instead. The head midwife was supportive of my decision and said its only a 1% risk- let's not think about that. She also explained that I would feel a different pain if the scar was thinning so I ensured throughout the labour that I kept a focus on the scar and if I felt any twinge or tingling there – which thankfully I never did.

At 4 am I was cheeked again and found to be still at 4 cms. I was so disappointed and then they started the talk of rupturing membranes etc and I had a frightening conversation about anaesthesia should I need it as I had been very ill after previous anaesthesia.

In the end it was suggested that if I needed a section, I would have to be given an general anaesthetic. Well you can imagine the shock. We agreed that that was something I would never get over and so my notes were taken out again to write in that I had said I would prefer to have a reaction to the drugs and be sick for days afterwards than be given a general anaesthetic. At this stage I was sent to walk the halls! I was on the verge of tears, seeing my birth messed up again.

After my second walk the midwife told me not to get stressed by this but I told her that was too late, I already was. We walked again and when I came back, the head midwife came into chat to me and said she had decided I wasn't in established labour and was sending me off to the labour ward instead. This was such a relief and I was so thankful to the midwife for having the sense to see this and send me packing at 6am .

So off I was sent to he labour ward and given a shot of Pethadine to help me sleep.

I did manage to sleep and my husband went home to come back in again at 10am That morning I woke somewhat refreshed and relieved to be given some breathing space. When the doctors came on their rounds the consultant decided that we should have a plan and I reluctantly agreed that if nothing happened by 6pm I would have my waters broken and see what happens then. At this stage I thought, I'd agree as hopefully things would be moving by then and if I wasn't happy with the decision at 6pm, I could have that conversation then.

Less stress was best at this stage. About an hour later however, the registrar whom I'd met in the clinic and found very open to my discussions etc arrived into me and said that she had spoken with another consultant on duty and he had agreed that if I didn't want any intervention, there was no need to break my waters at 6. We'll, that was a weight off my shoulders. I thanked her and will always remember her intervention.

So, with this decision taken, it was agreed that I could move into the pre natal ward. I was slowly moving back out of the hospital!
In the pre natal ward the pressure was totally off, I could eat as I liked and wander around freely. No body was there watching me continuously. I took another shot of pethadine at 2pm and myself and my husband slept together on the bed for about 1.5 hrs. Afterwards I had a bath and rang my mum to let her know what was happening.

At 8pm My husband headed off home and when he was gone I decided to take another bath. In the end I stayed there for three hours and was cheeked every so often as I felt that the surges were getting stronger and maybe closer together. I enjoyed these few hours by myself with nobody watching me and for each surge I poured water over my belly and used the word 'relax' as a focus for my breathing, breathed in Reeee and out Laaax

My legs were tense and I shook them easily in the bath which helped release the tension. Eventually at 1am I decided to get out of the bath as I felt I needed my TENS machine, I timed my surges and found that they were now about 3-5 minutes apart. I had the machine put on and then asked to be examined. I was 7 cms and being sent back to the delivery ward. The midwife wanted to wheel me over but I was more comfortable walking. I rang my husband to come in. I walked down to the delivery suite and the two midwives from the previous night were there and they gave me a round of applause saying 'we were wondering when you were going to come back to us!'

So I was settled into room four and I rang my husband again who had fallen back asleep. I think he got a fright when I said I was in the delivery room! Another trace was put on and all was well and I got hooked up to the gas and air – I LOVE that stuff!!!! When My husband arrived I relaxed and we listened to great music they had piped into the room,

I swayed to David Bowie singing 'Let's Dance' and we both danced together and laughed and thought about opening a bar where entonox is piped into it. There was a lovely intimate and somewhat romantic atmosphere. The two midwives came in and out and left us to it until about 5am when they decided to check and see where we were at. The waters still hadn't broken and I was starting to breathe differently and almost feel like bearing down but not quite. When I was checked the midwife felt a lip of cervix was still there and she thought it would help if she broke my waters. At this stage I was happy for them to be broken as I wanted some of the pressure relieved and a was a little bit anxious as this was the stage where my last labour ended up in a section. Once I felt the warm swoosh of water, everything started to change and the baby's head started to descend.

Before this however, I had a short while where everything stopped while we waited for something to happen. It was quite relaxing as we all sat there waiting.

Once the second stage started, there was no mistaking it! The midwives encouraged me into upright positions. I started initially in the chair and then to kneeling against the back of the chair. I didn't like this position though, I found the sensations so powerful and initially I spent more time concentrating on trying to get away from them. It was like I was trying to scramble away from an animal that had suddenly been let loose inside me. This stage was like nothing I could ever have imagined. There was no pain whatsoever but the power was incredible. My husband tells me that he never heard me make the sounds I did during this stage, they were so guttural. It's interesting because throughout this stage the image of a lion kept popping into my head and between surges I would lie back and say things like Gosh, Goodness Gracious. I found the pushing tiring and I did try at times to pretend I wasn't having a surge so that I would get a break but they knew what I was up to! Even My husband mentioned it afterwards, he could se that I had been pretending not to have them!

The midwives were great at relaxing me and getting me to focus on relaxing my bottom and focusing on bearing down. I needed their coaching and My husband was great with the affirmations at this stage reminding me to release and relax and that there was a wide open space for which my baby to descend. I did put on my headphones at one stage but soon tore them off, I found them too distracting and I felt like I needed to listen to the midwives. During one particular surge I felt what seemed like a couple of cracks internally, the midwives told me at this time that I was opening well and I knew that this was the sensation of the baby's head moving though my pelvis.
At each surge My husband and the midwives reassured me and congratulated me when I opened more. I was very hot and My husband kept me cooled down with a cold flannel. My legs were

very tense and the midwives massaged then between surges before placing them back on their hips for each surge.

Eventually, I was told they could see the baby's head, the midwives took my hand so that I could feel his head and knowing he was this close really helped me concentrate and focus on pushing. Eventually, the head emerged and I could see the baby lying sideways. The next push and the body slithered out, what a relief. It was popped up on my chest and I checked to see if it was a boy or a girl. A little boy – our Daniel Evan had arrived.

The third stage was managed and I found it tiring having to think about anymore pushing. The placenta was bigger than the midwives had ever seen, weighing over 1 kg. All during this time I had the baby on my chest, he was never taken from me and he had his first feed for about 20 mins before being taken to be weighed etc. He weighed 9lbs 9oz and was alert immediately. When I focused on the music that was playing I realised it was Leonard Cohen singing Hallelujah. How appropriate! Even though I had my own playlist, the music the hospital had piped into the room all the way through was perfect.

I had a small external tear as he came out with his hand up and this had to be sutured without anaesthesia. (I was thankful I had done my perineal massage for the last six weeks especially as I had pushed instead of breathing down).For the first time in the whole process I felt pain and no amount of sucking on gas and air dulled that pain. I gave the poor doctor such evil looks and my husband tells me my language was quite colourful.

Afterwards, I felt weak and the shower took a lot out of me. It's incredible how we can be so powerful one minute and wiped out the next. On my return I tucked into my tea and toast before being sent off to the bed which would be mine for the next three days with my son. A beautiful experience and one which so many people played a part in.

▌ VBAC after Two Caesareans

My first pregnancy in 2004 went very well, although the scan put his due date about one week ahead of my own dates. I didn't think much of it and as the EDD came and went I was booked for induction at 40+7. I knew nothing of the risks and was looking forward to meeting my baby.

Only 20 minutes or so after induction with pessaries my son was getting decelerations. The obs team were already in theatre so I was brought down for caesarean. My beautiful son was born and stitched and sore I forgot about the birth and focussed on my new baby.

My next pregnancy in 2006 I desperately wanted a natural VBAC, I thought I was supported but again the scan put my due date one week ahead. For a VBAC I was told I would have to come straight in with early labour for constant monitoring and I could not be induced. Again my EDD came and went and I was booked for a caesarean section for 40+8. I argued desperately for more time as I was having strong Braxton hicks I was told if I refused the planned caesarean they would not help me when I did go into labour...

My son was born 7lb 11oz, he was beautiful and fed straight away but I was told that after two caesareans vaginal birth would be impossible and worried about having more children. In the year that followed I was prompted to look into the possibility of VBAC2. At first I thought I was mad but I found that it was done and was a safe option.

The groups www.VBAC.co.uk, www.ICAN-online.org, www.caesarean.org.uk. Were full of inspirational women and their stories and in 2008/09 they helped me through my next pregnancy with info, info, info.

I was still unsure of what to do as all this support was only online.

My first cons app in UCHG was difficult, there was crying, shouting and high emotions in the room. The cons insisted I could not go for VBAC2, and that no Doctor would "allow" it and was full of false stats. By Irish law the hospital had to provide care, and the forcing surgery on any woman was against the convention of human rights. I told him that I would not consent to an unnecessary caesarean but if it became necessary I would reconsider my options. He looked at my notes and felt both my caesareans had been unnecessary, we agreed a birth plan together: monitoring with freedom of movement, vaginal examinations would be no more then 2 hourly, no syntocin drip, ARM etc. I also felt I had to lie about my due date putting it one week later then I knew it was to take the pressure off me if I went over.

My fantastically supportive pregnancy yoga instructor encouraged me to meet with one of the Midwives, a great woman supportive of VBAC2 she told me that ruptures were extremely uncommon and did not occur in early labour so I could safely stay home until around 5cm to avoid intervention. Also that the Royal College of surgeons recommends VBAC2 for all suitable women and that this is safe. (this report can be viewed on their website). My cons wished me luck. I was ready.

The pains /rushes started sometime on the Sunday night around 11pm they came through the night and into the morning with some vomiting etc. My husband stayed home to mind the kids. Time went by very quickly but I was comfortable, happy and getting plenty of rest. Around 4pm I spoke on the phone to the Midwife we had met before, she knew I was worried about coming in too early and interventions so she said she would wait at the hospital and examine me herself. We headed in and after a few walks around UCHG car park we went in and I was examined at 6.30pm I was 3-4cm and was happy to stay in. My pains slowed a bit in hospital at first but I was reassured this was normal. A lovely Midwife held the monitor on my belly to get a good trace as I walked, rocked and moved on the ball. I spent a lot of time off the monitor taking the long route to and from the toilet as often as possible, and ate and drank freely. I was coping well and happy although a bit loud.

I was examined again around 8.50pm, I was 5cm hurray I was progressing so no need to call the Doctor. 10 mins or so later and the pains started to change. I very suddenly felt I couldn't cope, I knew that an epidural would probably mean a repeat caesarean. I felt broken and lost. It never crossed my mind that this could be transition. Around 9.20 my waters broke as I was asking/BEGGING for an epidural. My Midwife asked me if I felt like I need to push, still thinking I was around 5cms I thought she was mad and began to tell her this when I was interrupted by a huge contraction and I felt my baby moving down, and started to panic. A second Midwife came in and I was encouraged onto the bed on all fours, at around 9.25/9.30. I was 10cms!

I tried the gas and air but found I couldn't use it. Not much was happening for a few minutes except me panicking. My husband and Midwife snapped me out of it and I got my breath back under control. She moved all the way through me with one big contraction, another and her head was out, I felt her wiggle and turn, it was a fantastic feeling! She was out and perfect.

I reached down and picked her up. It was 9.36pm. Everything had gone so quick I was a bit shocked. I needed a few stitches but all was well and we were happily transferred to the postnatal ward. The next day my daughter began to get unwell she was brought up to NICU, an ovarian cyst that had been seen on her scan actually turned out to be a cyst in her duodenum obstructing it. I followed her to Crumlin hospital and slept on the floor beside her cot for her surgery and recovery. I know that had I have had a caesarean it would not have been as easy for me to care for her during that difficult 2 weeks. Thankfully she had a full and quick recovery.

I look back on the moment of birth of all my children with joy, but with my daughter the whole day and birth experience was wonderful, and I can't believe it's been almost a year since that day.

So if your still with me this far, yes you can do it, yes it is safe and yes it's 100% worth it.

Gail's 3 Homebirths after a Caesarean

My first child was due early Nov 1997, I was only 22 and hadn't much clue about pregnancy and birth but it was in my head from an early age that I would have a natural, "easy" birth, no epidural and maybe Pethidine if necessary. From about 30 weeks I was told he was breech and the plan was to wait and see if he turned and if not the doctor would try ECV, and I pushed him to allow me a "trial of labour" if that didn't work.

However, when I was visiting my family in Tipperary at 36 weeks my waters broke! I live in Drogheda so I considered travelling back up but then thought better not chance it and went into Limerick Maternity. They loved me there, unbooked, unmarried and telling them the baby was breech!! I was admitted and told I would have a scan in the morning to see if it was breech! During the night I started getting mild contractions and don't remember sleeping much.

In the morning I had my scan and I think he may have been transverse at that stage although I wasn't told anything, just that the doctor would see me later. When she came around she said I would be having a caesarean today, no questions asked. There was no scope for discussion, that was it and I could like it or lump it. So, of course I didn't put up much of a fight. While waiting for the op I was getting stronger contractions and I remember when the trolley came for me at about 3 the ward sister was giving out to the staff that I was obviously labouring and should have been in theatre sooner. I was never examined so I don't know if I was dilated much but the relief I felt from the spinal makes me think I was probably in active labour.

The operation itself was fine, my partner, Will, just made it down from Drogheda to see our son being born, my Mam was on stand-by to come in if he didn't make it. He was absolutely amazed by the birth and the doctor holding Aaron up after she took him out. I felt great until the anaesthetist gave me something after he was born, and I became so groggy then and really don't remember much of the next 12 hours or so. I have a vague memory of holding him for a short while but don't know if I breastfed him or who was minding him at all. I didn't bond very well with him in the first few weeks and I have always blamed that on the drug I was given.

In the middle of that night 2 midwives got me out of bed and onto the toilet where my catheter came out and I made sure to get up and move about plenty after that. Breastfeeding took off pretty well despite him getting cup feeds and I think one or two bottles on the 1st and 2nd nights.

On the Monday, when he was 3 days he had to be admitted to Special Care as they thought he might have a bowel infection. He had to fast for 2 days which was very hard on all of us and he had IV antibiotics. I pumped to keep up my supply and luckily when he was allowed feed again he took to it no problem, even though he'd had a soother for the 2 days. At 6 days I was discharged from the ward but was able to stay in a room in the SCN until he was discharged at 9 days. Will was even allowed stay with me one night as I was very tearful.

All in all, the experience was a good one. I don't remember feeling cheated of my natural birth. I suppose I just went with the flow, and did what I was told but I was ok with that. It was still a time when you didn't question much, the doctor is always right! And if I was having my 1st baby now, and he was breech I think I would probably opt for a section unless I could be guaranteed a very skilful midwife or doctor was available for a vaginal birth.

A couple of weeks after he was born when we were back at home in Drogheda, I started to pass very big clots. I was admitted to OLOL with possible infection. I there a couple of days and the clots were still coming so I was brought back to theatre. The consultant found that a very small piece of placenta was left in my uterus. I was then on antibiotics also and of course Aaron and I ended up getting thrush.
The 1st 6-8 weeks of his life are a blur really because of major surgery, feeding, blood loss, lack of sleep!! I stopped breast-feeding at about 6 weeks which really disappointed me as I had plans for doing it for months. And I had to go back to work when he was only 14 weeks. When I think of it now I don't know how I did it, it's a good thing he was my first!

Our next birth was a wonderful homebirth. I believed that being at home would offer me the best chance to have a vaginal birth. I knew from working in the hospital that as soon as I'd be in the door I'd be considered high-risk and I felt I was no-where near high risk. I didn't want continuous monitoring, an IV or any pressure to perform in a certain time limit. Also I didn't want any pain relief to mask any potential problems and I would be more likely to take it if it was easily available. As it happened I would gladly have had an epidural with Liam if the anaesthetist had turned up at my house offering one, but the thoughts of the car journey felt like a tougher option at the time!! Obviously, I'm very glad I didn't have one. So essentially to start off with the homebirth wasn't my goal, a vaginal birth was what I really wanted and felt I was capable of-it and it just happened that home was the best place to achieve that. Since having one homebirth though I'd never consider hospital again unless there was a real obstetric need for it.

▌ Our last wonderful homebirth

I thought after our 3rd child I'd definitely never go again, I suffered from mild depression which responded well to acupuncture and I'd had a good bit of pain with SPD which got worse with each pregnancy. But I also remember saying if I ever had another I'd leave a bigger gap between them. So when David was about 3 and a half I got pregnant again. I found almost immediately I was very nauseous which lasted until about 15 weeks, luckily there wasn't much vomiting. It stopped and I had one week of feeling good when the SPD kicked in again, this time was much earlier and more severe. I had a few sessions of osteopathy which helped a little and managed to work with difficulty up to 27 weeks. I saw a physio then who gave me crutches and it helped but only if I walked really slowly. I had difficulty on the stairs, getting from sitting to standing, driving and even shopping as I couldn't manoeuvre a trolley. It was a very difficult time and I made sure to have photo evidence of it in case I ever felt broody again!!!

This time we couldn't have Dolores as our midwife as she was retiring in August and I was due the 26th of December. We were very disappointed but found a great replacement in Susan. She gave us the same care as Dolores, wonderful, relaxed visits at home and great patience with the kids. Like Dolores she was not too happy to do waterbirths which was fine with me, it would have been nice but not an absolute essential. She has great knowledge of homeopathy so had me on a regime from early on of different tissue salts and was fine with me not wanting any scans. We kept a good record of the pregnancy with photos, video and Will did a belly cast for me. And on Halloween night he painted my stomach to look like a pumpkin, it was brilliant, so life-like.

As I had been early with all the others I was full sure this little one would be just as obliging. I had great plans to be all done for Christmas. Also, a big family gathering was planned for

Friday the 28th for my grandmothers 80th birthday and I was not going to miss that. Little did I know!! Like with the others I had strong Braxton Hicks contractions for a few weeks towards the end and each night I imagined this will be it. But nothing. Then coming up to Christmas I started wanting it after the 28th as I didn't think a Christmas baby would thank us in years to come. Around the 24th my pelvis began to improve, so on the 26th we decided to go for our usual Stephens Day walk. I started off ok around a local wood but half way I could barely move and I hadn't brought the crutches. Will offered to carry me but that would have been a bit difficult! So he found 2 long sticks and I managed to hobble back to the car and I didn't venture out again.

On the 27th my sister and her boyfriend arrived over from England for the 80th party, they stayed in a B&B in Drogheda. I kind of hoped I'd labour that night so she could have been there to see it but I also wanted to hold off to get to the party. The next day my parents and brother arrived, en route to the party also, and stayed a few hours. I noticed a few twinges while they were here but said nothing and when they left we were still planning on seeing them all later that evening.

I went for a rest around 4 and was still feeling mild, irregular tightenings. At 5.30 I got up and called Will from the top of the stairs and said we should maybe head up to the hotel now (about 45 mins away) and just stay for a little while. As I stood there in a top and knickers he asked had I wet myself! I looked and saw sure enough my knickers were damp. I went to the loo and more fluid drained but unlike with the boys it was just a small bit, so I was a bit unsure. But within a short space the tightenings got more regular and stronger so we reckoned we'd have to miss the party. Typical, after waiting so long she decided to come when she wanted to.

So it was action stations again. I had promised our son Liam we would make the baby a birthday cake so we set about doing that and Will did some tidying up in the birth room. I had to stop about every 5 mins or so to hold onto the wall or the counter and breathe through the pains, which were manageable. I rang Susan and said I reckoned it would be tonight but didn't need her just yet. Around 7 they got a bit stronger again so I rang her back and she said she'll head over. I got the cake cooked and made a lovely lemon, sugar and honey drink for the labour as I wasn't hungry. I rang Sinead who was coming again as babysitter/doula. I got annoyed with Will over something and we had a bit of a row so when Susan arrived around 8.30 I was in the bedroom crying. She came up, calmed me and asked to examine me. I was 3cms and delighted with that so I got over my annoyance with Will fairly quickly. Sinead arrived around 9.30, and I was downstairs walking between the kitchen and the birth room as Will filled the pool and Susan got all her bits ready. I was surprised with all the equipment she had, a lot more than Dolores as I remember.

Around 10.30 or 11 the pool was ready and I got in. It was nice but not as good a feeling as I had on the others. I felt my position wasn't right, I was better standing leaning against the wall, but as Will had spent so long getting it ready I felt I better look like I appreciated it. I stayed in for about 20 mins and we have photos of me smiling with the boys standing around me which I love.

I started feeling some pressure so got out to stand again, but the pressure felt like needing to push without the real urge which I was used to. I wasn't sure what to do and probably panicked a bit. I tried kneeling and standing, and Susan suggested lying down which I wouldn't do. Then she asked could she examine me so I lay on the couch, I was 9 and a half cms. She asked me to lie on my side for a few minutes which was excruciating, Will told me after that I pulled hairs from his leg through his jeans!

Then suddenly I got a proper urge and felt the baby move right down through me, it was amazing. I jumped up off the couch, back onto all fours shouting "its coming now". Susan got ready and soon she could see the head which went back up just a couple of times before coming right out. All this we got on video which I am so glad of, it is so lovely to look back on once in a while. Sinead was doing it first, when Susan asked her to get some towels, so she handed it to Aaron (10) who managed to get amazing footage and cheer me on at the same time. It seemed like a lifetime waiting after the head was born until the rest of her came but she did eventually, at 00.02, and the cheers that went up were fantastic. Susan showed Will she was a girl and he told me. I was so shocked, I really thought she'd be another boy.

Susan handed her straight through to me and all the boys got a good look. Aaron and Liam (6) watched the birth and David (4) stayed just outside the door, coming in as soon as she was born and he cut her cord when it stopped pulsating (which he had decided from early on was to be his job). They got me and the baby all sorted and tucked up in the sofabed and we had a lovely cup of tea and toast. Then I rang my Mam at the party which Sinead got on video and you can hear the huge cheer there as the news got out. Susan checked the baby and she weighed 7lbs 14ozs, almost a pound lighter than the last which was fine with me! We called her Kate, after Wills mother and granny and my Nana (who died earlier that year), and Maria after my Mam Mary and Nana Maura. Susan stayed a few hours sorting everything out. I contemplated keeping the placenta but as we hadn't any of the boys ones it didn't seem right to keep only hers. She breastfed beautifully and we managed 4 months which I was very proud of.

Again the aftercare for homebirths is second to none, it was lovely seeing Susan regularly over the next 2 weeks and I was sad to see her go. We have been in touch a few times since but only work related, not to ask for her services again! Kate is my last and even as I type this 2 and a half years later I am not broody, a little nostalgic for the whole experience, but not enough to do it again. I've definitely hung up me boots this time!!!

▌ Optimising your Chances of a Positive VBAC

First off—take care of yourself—no big surprises here—being in good shape and eating well makes a VBAC more likely. The healthier you are both emotionally and physically the better.

Line up your VBAC team—I can't stress this strongly enough—if your last consultant/hospital's policies contributed to your first caesarean (i.e. routine induction). They may not support your choice of VBAC (or perhaps in a limited capacity). As you read in Mama's VBAC diary many health providers pay lip service to VBACs but in reality are not keen on them and will put so many limits on your labour that it will be very hard to have a VBAC.

When Planning a VBAC in Ireland there are basically 3 philosophies of care for VBAC in hospital. As you read through the list it will become quite obvious which philosophy your caregiver has. VBAC expert Jennifer Kamel discusses these 3 very different approaches and how they can impact your decision to have a VBAC.

1. The Doctor who says he doesn't support VBAC. This can be disappointing especially if you have a previous relationship with him/her. But this declaration is actually a good thing—you know exactly where you stand with him. Better you find out now right at the beginning so you can find a Doctor that will support you. At least he's being upfront and there won't be any nasty surprises at 38 weeks. You can change to public care or consider an out of hospital birth with a self employed community midwife.

2a. What's even more annoying is when the support is conditional on you being a good patient. First off they will say yes they are supportive *but* unless you are a particular star sign and can trace your ancestry back to the Stone Age their support is conditional. Jennifer Kamel calls this a "circus act VBAC."

They want you to think that if you just jump through all these hoops, you will have a VBAC. But what you don't know is that it's almost impossible to meet the standard they require and, one way or another, you'll probably end up with another surgery.

- if your baby is less than X pounds

- if you consent to continuous external, or internal, fetal monitoring

- if you stay in bed the whole time

- if you come to the hospital as soon as labour begins

- if you have the baby within X hours of labour starting

- if you have the baby within X hours of your water releasing

- if you agree to have a caesarean scheduled at X weeks "just in case" you don't go into labour

- if you agree to have an epidural

- if you agree to be induced at X weeks

- if you go into labour by X weeks and if you don't, you agree to have another caesarean or be induced

- it goes on, and on, and on...

2b. Or they tell you that they are supportive, but as your due date gets closer, they start focusing more and more on the risks of VBAC. Of course, they minimize, or don't even mention, the risks of having a repeat caesarean. It eventually becomes clear to you that they will find some excuse either during your labour, or before labour begins, to schedule a caesarean. At this point, how can you trust their medical opinion? But, they have strung you along for so long—usually this starts in the last couple months of your pregnancy—that you feel stuck and you think that it's too late to find another consultant. Sometimes it is, and sometimes it isn't. It never hurts to check out other consultants, regardless of how far along you are. When you have a Doctor like this, what do you have to lose?

3. The smallest group of care providers out there are the ones who are truly supportive of VBAC.

It is critical to carefully research and understand VBAC issues and choose your hospital/Doctor/Midwife accordingly. You must also be willing to consider switching Doctors/Midwives or go public if you are faced with a 'bait & switch' situation as you approach full term.

A Doctor or Midwife who is 'willing to let you try' is not good enough—if you go private you want a caregiver who expects that you WILL have a successful VBAC. Many hospitals still consider VBAC Mums as having a 'trial of scar' or a 'trial of labour.' Jennifer maintains "The VBAC mother needs acknowledgment and support, not criticism and judgment. She and her uterus are not---must not be---on 'trial.' "

Although finding a truly supportive and non-interventive provider can be challenging, the process of educating yourself, trusting your gut, and searching for a compatible provider is a vital and dynamic part of preparing for a different and better birth. Don't let the naysayers get you down; consider it part of the journey.

Take some time to find a supportive Doctor or Midwife, his VBAC rate should be at least 70% and get support from other VBAC Mums. It's a great idea to do this research before you get pregnant—that way all of your ducks are in a row when you get those two lines and you can relax and enjoy your pregnancy. Homebirth may also be an option for you.

You will hear from some caregivers and even friends/family members that the main goal is a healthy baby and Mum. This infers that the goal of VBAC and the goal of a healthy baby are incompatible. This is not an either or situation........"Mrs Byrne you can have the positive birth experience you're insisting on OR a healthy baby" This sounds like a planned caesarean guarantees a healthy Mum and baby...it doesn't—in most cases it's *less* safe. What normal woman would chose a VBAC if she thought she was putting her baby at risk? According to Gina a UK VBAC campaigner "A caesarean mother would never put her baby at risk—she will always make the sacrifice she has made before if there is the slightest indication that it will benefit her baby. The baby always comes first, the birth experience second". As a Mother or Father reading this book you know Mothers do not go against medical advice lightly.

▌ Monitoring Your Baby During VBAC

It is routine practice to monitor your baby continuously as there have been very few studies on VBAC and continuous monitoring versus VBAC and intermittent monitoring.

The available research suggests that continuous foetal monitoring catches the *most consistent* signs of scar separation—but that doesn't mean it's the only sign—other signs would be changes to the pattern of your surges, drop in your blood pressure, slower heart rate in your baby, Mother's pulse changes, pain and maybe bleeding. There are reports in the research of Mums experiencing scar separation without any pain. But if you think about it logically if a Mum starts to loose blood her pulse would be affected—the CTG only picks up the problem in your baby when blood flow is compromised to your baby...... which is after the fact. Would it make more sense for a mothers pulse to be more closely monitored instead?

VBAC is one of the situations when the medical literature supports the use of continuous EFM. The sad irony is that it's the misuse of the CTG that probably contributed to Mum having her caesarean in the first place. But VBAC experts say that this is not necessarily a reason to "require" continuous fetal monitoring since it hasn't been shown to improve outcomes even in VBACs. Catching a scar separation right away is important, but it's the difference in outcomes that we need to be looking for.

It is ultimately your choice —hopefully you can reach a compromise with the hospital so everyone is happy. Ask about using a telemetry CTG (it's wireless so you can be mobile). In some maternity units part of their 'management' plan is to break your waters and attach a monitor to your baby's scalp. This is very invasive and routine breaking the waters introduces more risks and according to the most recent Cochrane research it can increase your risk of having another caesarean but some Mums see it as a trade off for the freedom to be mobile and not stuck to the bed for monitoring so they manage their labour easier. Being confined to the bed during the birth process means you're more likely to need an epidural as you can't move about/use the bath etc and as we know the epidural can sometimes slow labour which means you're more likely to need acceleration with synthetic oxytocin which then makes foetal distress more likely and/or problems with the scar integrity. Remember 'true' scar separation is extremely rare.

If you do have continuous (external) monitoring ask your Midwife to give you the telemetry unit—it's a wireless CTG so you can be up and moving around.

▌ I Want To Stay Home Longer In Labour—Is It Safe?

This is the million dollar question and a somewhat controversial one. Most VBAC Mums acknowledge that being able to stay home in their own surroundings and labour without the distractions and stress of the hospital is important. As soon as you get to hospital you're on the clock and on the CTG (unless you've negotiated intermittent monitoring). Labouring at home when planning a VBAC might be safer than spending that time labouring in hospital in the same ways that having a planned out of hospital birth generally compares very favourably to hospital birth. Some Irish VBAC friendly Doctors tell Mums not to be in a huge hurry in to the hospital when labour gets started.

Labouring in the comfort of your own home you and your baby's safety is increased in some ways by not having routine interventions (breaking your waters, speeding up your labour, induction, epidurals, assisted birth and of course infections). Unfortunately there have been no studies comparing labouring at home or HBAC (homebirth after caesarean). We know that the risks are higher once you've had a caesarean whether you plan a repeat caesarean section or a VBAC—and it's hard to quantify without research how staying home for longer might be of benefit. But it seems like a no brainer to be in the place where you're going to labour most efficiently and with the least amount of stress.

Ultimately you'll need to determine where you'll feel safer and what makes most sense for you and your circumstances. Some Mums will feel safer being at the hospital right from the beginning. Weigh up the pros and cons and decide what works for you on the day.

▓ I Would Like to labour in a Birth Pool and/or have a Waterbirth

The use of warm water in labour is well documented for having significant benefits for the Mother including reducing her need for augmentation (speeding up of labour) and epidurals. Most Mothers using warm water are very satisfied with their labour experiences. Currently waterbirth is only available at home with a self employed community Midwife (hopefully this will change in the future). Labouring in water (baby is born on dry land) is only an option in the two Midwife Led Units in the North East but currently this option is only available to low risk Mums. Mothers who have had a previous caesarean are not eligible.

It is expected that CUMH will open it's pool by mid Summer 2010 so it'll be up to VBAC Mums to request use of the pool.

In a UK VBAC (MIDIRS 2006) audit conducted by Dianne Garland, Mums who used birth pools had a VBAC rate of approx 88%. Monitoring of the fetal is with water Dopplers, listening in every 15 minutes or so. Mum's observations of temperature, pulse and blood pressure and one-to one care in labour are the guidelines.

▌ Questions to Ask about VBAC

Learn all you can about your hospital policies for VBAC—do they have time limits? (to avoid a Cinderella VBAC).

How negotiable is their policy on monitoring your baby during labour?

Will you have an opportunity to use a labour pool or the bath?

What happens if you go past your guess date?

What is their policy around induction/acceleration of a VBAC labour?

What is their policy on doulas or additional birth partners for support?

▌ Ways to Stack the Odds in Your Favour of VBAC

Ignore anyone who undermines your intention to have a VBAC.

If you're reading through the books or research whenever you see 'trial of labour' or 'trial of scar' mentally replace those words with 'opportunity to birth'. Change UR to scar separation. Remember 'true' UR is a very rare occurrence.

Write out your birth priorities and discuss them with your partner and your hospital/Midwife.

Take a class that will boost your confidence in normal birth such as GentleBirth or Cuidiu's classes or start using the GentleBirth CDs at home.

Read lots of positive VBAC stories and if your partner isn't completely on board consider having a Doula to keep you focused and positive. Your partner may still be coming to terms with the trauma of an emergency caesarean.

Connect with other VBAC Mums (see resources).

█ **What are the Risks if I've Already Had A VBAC?**

In a 2008 study (Mercer) concluded that the risk of scar separation drops 50% after the first VBAC.

▓ What If I've Had More than One Caesarean—is VBAC an Option?

If you've had more than one caesarean and would like an opportunity for a normal birth be prepared for a long road ahead
(especially if you try to convince your consultant to give you
a chance at VBAC) Planned VBAC2 doesn't happen often in
Ireland—when it happens it's generally accidentally rather than
being a planned and supported birth experience. Unless you
know that your consultant is 110% supportive of VBAC2 some
VBAC Mums suggest taking the path of least resistance...and
don't mention it until their last trimester. It's easier to deal with
2 or 3 weeks of negotiations than 9 months of fighting for an
opportunity to give birth normally.

In June 2006 the first comprehensive study was published that looks
at VBAC after multiple sections. The study included 18,000 women
over 4 years at 19 medical centres, comparing VBAC in those with 1
prior section to VBAC in those with multiple prior caesarean births.
Ruptures occurred in .7% of those with 1 prior section and .9% of
those with multiple caesareans. This is a negligible difference.

Some good news for VBAC Mums that came out of the UK in
2010—new research suggests that women who deliver vaginally
after three or more caesareans have similar rates of success and
complications as those who undergo another elective caesarean, according to a study in the current issue of the International Journal
of Obstetrics and Gynaecology (Feb 2010).

Of the 860 women with three or more prior caesareans, 89 attempted a vaginal birth after caesarean (VBAC) and 771 elected
for a repeat caesarean. The study sample size was small because
it's difficult to find women who try -- or are allowed -- to give
birth vaginally after repeated caesareans.

■ VBAC isn't an Option—What Can I do to Make this Next Caesarean a More Positive Experience.

In the UK Professor Nick Fisk has started what he calls a "natural caesarean". This groundbreaking approach to surgical delivery — Fisk calls it a "skin-to-skin caesarean" or "walking the baby out" — has been pioneered by him partly in response to the rising caesarean rate. As Fisk started to examine the conventions of surgical delivery, he was struck by how easily they could be challenged. Why, for example, did they need to be done so quickly, when slowing them down would give the parents more chance to participate in their child's delivery and might give the baby a gentler experience of coming into the world? Why, too, was it so important for the parents to be screened off from the mother's abdomen? And was it really essential for the baby to be whisked off for an immediate medical examination, rather than delivered into the arms of his mother?

This is the birth of your child, a completely different surgical experience than any other, an experience to be treated as similarly to a vaginal birth experience as is humanly possible.

If you do need a caesarean, then it would be better for you to receive a spinal/epidural anaesthetic and remain conscious during the operation, participating in the birth of your child.

If an emergency caesarean is necessary under general anaesthetic, then be sure your baby is given to your partner as soon as possible after birth and held by him (hopefully next to his naked chest — skin to skin contact) until you are awake and can be told of the baby's sex and well-being (by your partner).

If an elective caesarean is necessary, then you should request that you be able to begin labour naturally before the caesarean is done. That is, you do not want a date and time preset; you wish for your baby to decide the day on which it is ready to be born to avoid any problems with prematurity and for both of you to reap the benefits of your hormones.

Your baby should remain with you at all times — no disappearing off to the nursery with your partner. No matter how "nice" this is, it can affect your bonding with your new baby. If your baby must go to the nursery, then do send your partner and encourage the "skin-to-skin" contact mentioned before. Your baby will really be craving this contact, and he will most likely recognise your partner's voice.

Make sure theatre staff realise that you would appreciate a verbal description of the birth as it occurs. You may have previously felt left out of your past caesarean(s) as your body and labour might have been discussed as though you weren't there.

How about asking the surgeon to leave the umbilical cord long and allow the father the chance to cut it? That way the parents do not miss out on the sensation or their own right to tell their story of "cutting a cord".

Would you like to meet your new baby in his/her unclothed, naked newborn state — a wet, slippery baby? Then request that the baby please be placed on your chest with a warm blanket over you both. It would do a lot to make this surgical delivery a bit more natural for mother, father and baby. And it may even resolve a few inner conflicts that are faced after the birth.

How about breastfeeding your baby straight away? Let them know that you would like to feed your baby while you are being sutured, if you feel up to it, and you would like your baby to stay with you throughout the surgery and even during the recovery. Or you could arrange for the lactation consultant of the hospital (or your own private one) to be present at the caesarean birth and bring the baby to you in recovery, to breastfeed within that first hour of birth.

Let them know that your partner would be delighted to hold his/her child within your view throughout these procedures, if you feel unable to participate in the bonding (at least you would be able to witness it this time).

You may also be able to organise with your Doctor to allow a quiet relaxation CD to be played throughout the birth. Don't let it intrude on the birth, though; just enough to gently enhance the experience.

What about that placenta? Most women who birth vaginally get to see it, at least, and maybe you would like to.

Make a birth plan! Have several copies with you and give it to everyone involved in your caesarean! They won't know what is important to you unless you let them know.

Write to the Head of Obstetrics in the hospital about your birth plan. That way, they have plenty of time to fully understand what you want, as well as give them the opportunity to raise with you any concerns they may have. Once you have both reached an agreement about your caesarean then get that agreement in writing and take it with you to the hospital so staff do not have to run around and "get approval" from the appropriate person.

Ask the hospital to take you through every step of the procedure. Make sure they explain to you every light and every sound. Much of the anxiety happens when you can see flashing lights and disturbing noises and you don't know what it means.

Make sure that there is someone to take digital photos of the birth and the baby (in case you are having a general anaesthetic). Then if the baby has to be taken away for observation you can see pictures of the baby as soon as you wake from the procedure. You can use a mobile phone but the quality won't be as good — but you can send it to friends and family immediately.

After being wheeled into the recovery room, ask that they dim the lights for you and your baby. (This might not be possible, especially if you have a few other patients in the recovery ward and checks requiring observations are being done all the time).

You might want a special blanket to wrap baby in while waiting with you at recovery. Note that if your baby is with you at recovery, most hospitals will require a Midwife to be in attendance. This is why it's a good idea to get the head of maternity and operating theatre involved very early, to assist with staffing requirements.

© Birthrites.com

▍When is VBAC Not Recommended?

According to the Royal College of Obstetricians and Gynecologists in the UK (2007) there are very few occasions when VBAC is not advisable and a repeat caesarean birth is likely to be the safer choice for you and your baby. These would include:

- If you have had three or more previous caesarean births (but see recent 2010 RCOG article about VBAC3)
- the scar has separated during a previous labour
- you have a high uterine incision (classical caesarean)
- you have other pregnancy complications that require a caesarean delivery.

▍Welcoming Your Baby

Caesarean or VBAC—whatever your decision (if you have a choice) always remember that this is the day you get to meet your baby. This is your baby's birthday—a day that you will never forget. It's a day that you will want to remember for all the right reasons and the more involved you can be in your own care the more satisfying the experience will be for you.

Wishing you a wonderful birth.

Tracy Donegan

RESOURCES

Big Babies (includes VBAC birth stories)
http://www.bigbaby.org.uk/vbacs_with_a_big_baby.html

Bereavement Support
Bereaved Parents Association, St Francis Day Hospital,
    Grange Road, Dublin 5; Tel: 01-8318788.
Irish Sudden Infant Death Association,
    4 North Brunswick Street, Dublin 7; Tel: 1850 391391;
    General Enquiries: 01-8732711.
The Miscarriage Association of Ireland,
    Carmichael Centre, North Brunswick Street, Dublin 7;
    Tel: 01-8735702. Fax: 8735737.

Birth Pool / Labour Pool
Mary Tighe – 0876-292 577

Birth Trauma Support
Anne Gill: Tel: 01-8450698.
AIMSIreland.com
Benig Mauger: www.soul-connections.com

Breastfeeding
La Leche League: http://homepage.eircom.net/~lalecheleague/
    help.html
Breastfeeding Clinic: www.breastfeeding-clinic.com.
    Enquiries to eileenosullivan@breastfeeding-clinic.com
www.ilca.org – for referrals to lactation consultants in Ireland
www.kellymom.com
Cuidiu (see below)

Cuidiu, The Irish Childbirth Trust
Cuidiu, Carmichael House, Brunswick Street, Dublin 7;
    Tel: 01-8724501, www.cuidiu-ict.ie

Caesarean / VBAC Support
ICAN: www.ican-online.org
ICAN Irish chapter: Tracy Donegan, Tel: 087-057-2500
Caesarean Support Group: 111 Wedgewood Maples, Sandyford, Dublin 16. Tel: 01-2954953
Sligo Caesarean Support Group: Gwen Scarbrough (Midwife); Tel: 087-6710985; www.informedbirthireland.com
Vaginal Birth after Caesarean: www.VBAC.com
AIMS Ireland – www.AIMSIreland.com
www.VBACFACTS.com
www.VBAC.org.uk

Doulas
Association of Irish Doulas: www.Doula.ie
Doula Ireland: www.doulaireland.com;
Tracy Donegan, Tel: 087-0572500.
Doula Information (UK): www.doula.org.uk
Doula Information (US): www.DONA.org

General Pregnancy/Parenting Websites
www.rollercoaster.ie
www.eumom.ie
www.thebabyorchard.com
www.mothering.com
www.babycenter.com
www.magicMum.com
www.WeddingsOnline.ie

Home Birth
The Homebirth Association of Ireland,www.homebirth.ie;
087-7533303 or enquiries@homebirth.ie

Holistic Practitioners
www.holisto.com
www.homeopathyireland.net

Hypnosis for Birth & Preparation for VBAC
GentleBirth – www.GentleBirth.ie

Informed Choices
www.infochoice.org
www.maternitymatters.org
www.motherfriendly.org
www.aims.org.uk
www.cochrane.org
www.childbirthconnection.org

Multiple Births
Irish Multiple Births Association: Carmichael House,
    North Brunswick Street, Dublin 7. Tel: 01 8749056.
    Email: info@imba.ie

Postnatal Depression
PND Association of Ireland: www.PND.ie;
    E-mail: support@pnd.ie
Aware, 72 Lower Leeson Street, Dublin 2; Tel: 01-6617211;
    Telephone helpline: 01-6766166, daily, 10.00 am – 10.00
    pm; Fax: (01) 6617217; E-mail: aware@iol.ie
Parentline, Carmichael House, North Brunswick Street,
    Dublin 7; Tel: 01-8787230; Helpline: 01-8733500; Email:
    parentline@eircom.net
Mental Health Ireland, Mensana House, 6 Adelaide Street,
    Dun Laoghaire, Co Dublin; Tel: 01-2841166;
    E-mail: info@mentalhealthireland.ie

Prenatal Parenting
www.birthpsychology.com
www.prenatalparenting.com

Single Parent Support
www.gingerbread.ie
www.solo.ie
www.treoir.ie

Yoga for Pregnancy
www.birthlight.com
www.yogapregnancy.net
www.yogaireland.com

Glossary

Active Management of Labour: Hospital guidelines for managing the birth process with time limits and routine interruptions to normal birth, originally implemented by the National Maternity Hospital in Dublin but carried out in most Irish maternity units.

Amniotic Fluid: The clear fluid that your baby floats in during pregnancy.

Amniotomy: See ARM

Apgar Score: Named after Virginia Apgar this is scoring system that evaluates your baby's adaptation to life outside the womb at 1 minute and at 5 minutes.

ARM (Artificial Rupture of Membranes): Your bag of waters are released artificially with an amnihook (looks like a crochet hook) instead of spontaneously.

Auscultation: To listen to your baby's heartbeat with a Pinard, Doppler or CTG.

Bishops Score: A rating system that may indicate the success of an induction.

Breaking the waters: See ARM

Breech: A baby that is presenting feet or backside first

Cardiotogography (CTG): A machine that monitors baby's heart rate (only recommended in high risk mothers)

Catheter: a thin tube that is inserted into the urethra to drain the bladder when you have an epidural. It can be left in if you have a caesarean.

Cervix: The opening to the uterus

Doula: A trained labour companion clinically proven to reduce caesarean rates and improve the mothers experience.

Eclampsia: A serious medical complication with seizures not attributed to another cause during pregnancy.

EDD: Estimated Due Date (Guess Date)

Entonox: A combination of gas and air used for pain relief in labour.

Epidural: A method of pain relief produced by an injection into the spine.

Episiotomy: An outdated surgical procedure involving cutting the perineal area to enlarge the vaginal opening

Evidence Based Care: Practices that are based on the best available clinical research

External Cephalic Version (ECV): A technique to manually turn a breech baby to a more favourable head down position

Foetal Distress: Reduction of oxygen to the baby, often indicated by consistent irregular heart rate

Forceps: An obstetric instrument used in assisted deliveries

GentleBirth: Antenatal birth preparation program using self hypnosis, visualisation and partner support techniques.

Hypertension: High blood pressure

Induction: The process of artificially starting labour

Kangaroo Care: Wearing your baby skin to skin

Kegels: Exercises to tone and strengthen the pelvic floor muscles

Lithotomy: Outdated birth position where Mother lies on her back

Membrane Sweep: A method of induction involving a vigorous internal examination to increase prostaglandin hormones.

Midwife: Caregiver specialising in normal birth

MLU: Midwife Led Unit

Moxibustion: A holistic therapy using heat and herbs, used to help positioning of posterior and breech babies.

Obstetrician: A Doctor specialising in abnormal and surgical birth

Oxytocin: A hormone generated by the brain that facilitates contraction of the uterus during birth and the milk ejection during breastfeeding. Also known as the 'mothering hormone'.

Pethidine: A narcotic drug used in labour for pain relief

Pinard: A tool used by Midwives for manually checking your baby's heartbeat intermittently

Placenta: An organ that develops in the uterus which sustains your baby during pregnancy.

Placental Abruption: A serious complication where the placenta comes away from the wall of the uterus prematurely causing bleeding.

Placenta Previa: A complication where the placenta can cover the cervix

PND: Post Natal Depression

Pre-eclampsia: A medical condition that occurs only during pregnancy and the postnatal period and affects both the mother and the baby. Swelling, sudden weight gain, headaches and changes in vision and high blood pressure are important symptoms.

Prolapse (cord): Complication, often caused by ARM, where the cord comes before the baby and is compressed, possibly resulting in foetal distress and caesarean.

Prostaglandin Gel: Artificial hormone that stimulates contractions of the uterus.

Sonicaid: A handheld electronic tool to check baby's heart rate

Syntometrine (aka Ergometrine, Syntocinon, Synthetic Hormone Oxytocin): Used to deliver the placenta in a managed third stage.

TENS (Transcutaneous Electrical Nerve Stimulation): Device used for pain management in labour

Transition: The point in labour when the cervix is between 8 and 10 cm dilated, where mothers often experience a lack of confidence.

Umbilical Cord: Your baby's connection to the placenta which carries oxygen and nutrients to you baby and waste way you're your baby.

Uterine Rupture: Scar separation occurring during pregnancy/birth.

VBAC: Vaginal Birth After Caesarean (i.e. for subsequent births)

Ventouse/Vacuum: An obstetric tool used for assisted deliveries

Vertex: Position of baby is head down

WHO: World Health Organisation

Recommended Reading

Crawford, Karis, *Natural Childbirth After Caesarean*

Donegan, Tracy, *The Better Birth Book 2006*. Liffey Press (Dublin)

Donegan, Tracy, *GentleBirth VBAC Preparation Program 2009* (Dublin)

Henci Goer, *The Thinking Woman's Guide to Better Birth*, 1999, Penguin (USA)

Hoy Angela, *Don't Cut Me Again*

Sears and Sears, *The Pregnancy Book*, 1997, Little, Brown (USA)

Ina May Gaskin's Guide to Childbirth, 2003, Bantam (USA)

Ina May Gaskin's Guide to Breastfeeding, 2009, (USA)

Dr Michel Odent, *The Caesarean*, 2004, Free Association Books, UK

Kim Wildner, *Mothers Intention: How Belief Shapes Birth*, 2003, Harbor and Hill (USA)

Benig Mauger, *Reclaiming the Spirituality of Birth*, 2000, Haling Arts (USA)

Granju and Kennedy, Attachment *Parenting: Instinctive Care for Your Baby and Young Child*, 1999 (USA)

Sarah J Buckley, *Gentle Birth, Gentle Mothering*, 2005, One Moon Press (Australia)

Nancy Wainer Cohen, *Open Season*, 1991, Bergin and Garvey (USA)